# KEY TOPICS IN
# CHRONIC PAIN
## SECOND EDITION

# The KEY TOPICS Series

Advisors:

**T.M. Craft** *Department of Anaesthesia and Intensive Care, Royal United Hospital, Bath, UK*
**C.S. Garrard** *Intensive Therapy Unit, John Radcliffe Hospital, Oxford, UK*
**P.M. Upton** *Department of Anaesthesia, Royal Cornwall Hospital, Treliske, Truro, UK*

Accident and Emergency Medicine, Second Edition
Anaesthesia, Clinical Aspects, Third Edition
Cardiovascular Medicine
Chronic Pain, Second Edition
Critical Care
Evidence-Based Medicine
Gastroenterology
General Surgery
Neonatology
Neurology
Obstetrics and Gynaecology, Second Edition
Oncology
Ophthalmology, Second Edition
Oral and Maxillofacial Surgery
Orthopaedic Surgery
Orthopaedic Trauma Surgery
Otolaryngology, Second Edition
Paediatrics, Second Edition
Psychiatry
Renal Medicine
Respiratory Medicine
Thoracic Surgery
Trauma

*Forthcoming titles include:*

Acute Poisoning
Cardiac Surgery
Cardio-Respiratory Physiotherapy
Clinical Research and Statistics
Urology

# KEY TOPICS IN
# CHRONIC PAIN
## SECOND EDITION

**Kate M. Grady**
**BSc, MB, BS, FRCA**
*Consultant in Anaesthesia and Chronic Pain Management,*
*South Manchester University Hospitals NHS Trust,*
*Manchester, UK*

**Andrew M. Severn**
**MA, MB, FRCA**
*Consultant in Anaesthesia and Chronic Pain Management,*
*Royal Lancaster Infirmary, Lancaster, UK*

**Paul R. Eldridge**
**MA, MChir, FRCS**
*Consultant Neurosurgeon,*
*Walton Centre for Neurology and Neurosurgery,*
*Liverpool, UK*

**Consultant Editor**

**Chris J. Glynn**
**MB, BS, DCH, FRCA, MSc**
*Churchill Hospital, Oxford, UK*

© BIOS Scientific Publishers Limited, 2002

First published 1997 (ISBN 1 85996 076 6)
Reprinted 1999
Second Edition 2002 (ISBN 1 85996 038 3)
Reprinted 2002, (twice)

ISBN 1 85996 038 3

BIOS Scientific Publishers Ltd
9 Newtec Place, Magdalen Road, Oxford OX4 1RE, UK
Tel. +44 (0)1865 726286. Fax +44 (0)1865 246823
World Wide Web home page: http://www.bios.co.uk/

Distributed exclusively in the United States, its dependent territories, Canada, Mexico, Central and South America, and the Caribbean by Springer-Verlag New York Inc, 175 Fifth Avenue, New York, USA, by arrangement with BIOS Scientific Publishers Ltd, 9 Newtec Place, Magdalen Road, Oxford OX4 1RE, UK.

**Important Note from the Publisher**
The information contained within this book was obtained by BIOS Scientific Publishers Ltd from sources believed by us to be reliable. However, while every effort has been made to ensure its accuracy, no responsibility for loss or injury whatsoever occasioned to any person acting or refraining from action as a result of information contained herein can be accepted by the authors or publishers.

The reader should remember that medicine is a constantly evolving science and while the authors and publishers have ensured that all dosages, applications and practices are based on current indications, there may be specific practices which differ between communities. You should always follow the guidelines laid down by the manufacturers of specific products and the relevant authorities in the country in which you are practising.

Production Editor: Nadine Séveno
Typeset by Jayvee Computer Services, Trivandrum, India
Printed by The Cromwell Press, Trowbridge, UK

# CONTENTS

[a] Contributed by A.F. Smith (FRCA, MRCP), Consultant Anaesthetist, Royal Lancaster Infirmary, Lancaster, UK.
[b] Includes contribution from B. Tait (FRACP, FFPM), Consultant Physician, Avenue Consultancy, Christchurch, New Zealand.

# ABBREVIATIONS

| | |
|---|---|
| AIDS | acquired immune deficiency syndrome |
| AVM | arteriovenous malformation |
| CABG | coronary artery bypass graft |
| CGRP | calcitonin gene-related peptide |
| CNS | central nervous system |
| COXIBs | cyclo-oxygenase II inhibitors |
| CPPWOP | chronic pelvic pain without obvious pathology |
| CPSP | central post-stroke pain |
| CRPS | complex regional pain syndromes |
| CSF | cerebrospinal fluid |
| CT | computed tomography |
| DMARD | disease-modifying antirheumatic drugs |
| DREZ | dorsal root entry zone |
| DSM | Diagnostic and Statistical Manual |
| EBM | evidence-based medicine |
| ESR | erythrocyte sedimentation rate |
| GABA | γ-amino butyric acid |
| HAD | hospital anxiety and depression index |
| HRT | hormone replacement therapy |
| IASP | International Association for the Study of Pain |
| IBS | irritable bowel syndrome |
| ICD | International Classification of Disease |
| LLLT | low-level laser therapy |
| MS | multiple sclerosis |
| MVD | microvascular decompression |
| NGF | nerve growth factor |
| NMDA | $N$-methyl-D-aspartic acid |
| NNH | number needed to harm |
| NNT | number needed to treat |
| NSAIDs | nonsteroidal anti-inflammatory drugs |
| PHN | post-herpetic neuralgia |
| PVD | peripheral vascular disease |
| RCT | randomized controlled trial |
| SIP | sympathetically independent pain |
| SLR | straight leg raise |
| SMP | sympathetically maintained pain |
| SSRI | serotonin specific re-uptake inhibitors |
| TCA | tricyclic antidepressants |
| TENS | transcutaneous electrical nerve stimulation |
| TGN | trigeminal neuralgia |
| THC | tetrahydrocannabinol |
| VSCC | voltage-sensitive calcium channels |
| WHO | World Health Organization |

# PREFACE TO THE SECOND EDITION

Four years after the publication of *Key Topics in Chronic Pain* it is time to ask what has changed. When we considered the invitation, the opportunity to modernize a few chapters was tempting, but we did not anticipate a complete revision.

The science of evidence-based medicine is evolving. Four years ago a few systematic reviews were easy to acquire, and relevant randomized controlled trials could be numbered. Now there are hundreds of each and we have had to be selective in choosing those which we believe are relevant to practice. We have therefore removed many references to randomized controlled trials in favour of systematic reviews. We have asked an expert to steer us through the conflicting principles of evidence-based medicine to allow us to publish treatments according to the quality of evidence afforded. At the same time we have kept an ear out for the respected colleagues who have valuable advice to offer on managing difficult problems. We have used the term 'it is reported that' or 'it is claimed that' for anecdotal, case report and uncontrolled observations, and the term 'it is shown that' or 'it is proven' for controlled trials. The last edition was designed specifically for the needs of postgraduate trainees in anaesthesia. This edition, we hope, will introduce the subject in a real way to other doctors, of all specialties and grades, and to nurses, therapists, psychologists and alternative practitioners.

The management of chronic pain is the science and art of rehabilitation. We believe that this concept sets apart legitimate approaches, by whomever they are practised, from less valuable treatments. There is pressure from all sides to respect opinions from a variety of sources, both 'conventional' and 'alternative'. It is not the function of this book to judge the various contenders for a rightful place in multidisciplinary practice, but it can at least set some rules by which practice can be judged.

Chronic pain remains a growing subspecialty, and its coexistence with the discipline of acute pain management is a relationship we are keen to promote. Hence the reader will find chapters on burn pain and pain during pregnancy, in the hope that a handy reference to taxing 'acute pain' problems will be available here.

The relationship between doctors, managers and their political masters has changed irrevocably in four years, and we have therefore made reference to this and the relationship of the pain clinician to the local community. By strange coincidence the day the manuscript was delivered to the publishers was also the day that Professor Patrick Wall died (8th of August 2001). Patrick Wall was a major influence on the philosophy of this book. His seminal 1965 paper with Ronald Melzack which described the 'gate control' theory of pain is an example of his influence. His direct personal encouragement of one of the authors and the opinions which he so eloquently expressed at scientific meetings and which have found their way into the text is another. We hope that in some measure through the text the spirit of Patrick Wall's challenging approach to the problems of patients with pain will be passed on to another generation of clinicians.

Our trainees have been at the forefront of our minds when writing this, and we are pleased to see many moving on to consultant posts around the world. We could not have started without the encouragement of Sara and Frank, and are privileged to welcome Paul Eldridge, a neurosurgeon, as an author. Andrew Smith, who is Editor of the Cochrane Anaesthesia Review Group, and Barrie Tait, a rehabilitation specialist, have contributed to the text. We also acknowledge the support of Jai Kulkarni, Michael Sharpe, Wendy Makin and Charles Cox for commenting on the manuscripts and Chris Glynn for his help in pulling the project together.

*Andrew Severn, Kathryn Grady*

# PREFACE TO THE FIRST EDITION

This latest volume in the Key Topics series aims to provide the health professional with up-to-date information about a range of issues in the management of chronic pain. It is not a substitute for the larger texts, nor is it an attempt to provide a comprehensive reference to palliative care or painful rheumatological and neurological conditions. It is a working manual of the common problems of management of the chronic pain sufferer, the patient in whom investigations have excluded treatable disease. The book is designed for specialist registrars, general practitioners, psychologists, nurses and physiotherapists. It is written by two hospital consultants responsible for running Pain Clinics in general hospitals, with two chapters provided by a colleague in a neurosurgical centre.

## What is chronic pain?

A definition that describes a chronic condition as a long-standing acute condition is inadequate. Tissues involved in chronic inflammation, for example, can be distinguished microscopically from those with acute inflammation by changes of regeneration and repair. Once a condition becomes chronic, secondary changes make for an immediate situation in which management involves treating complications of the condition rather than the condition itself. Thus it is with chronic pain. Chronic pain is not a symptom of an illness. It is an illness. It has its own symptoms, signs and complications. The professional caring for the chronic pain sufferer looks for complications of chronic pain and attempts to treat these. The original cause of the chronic pain may be irrelevant. If there is a possible cure the professional is advised to ascertain the degree to which the complications of chronic pain have become apparent: the complications themselves may seriously limit the benefit that might otherwise be obtained from treatment of the pain.

## This book

The opening chapters explain the terms with which the professional should be familiar, and some of the practical problems encountered in Pain Clinic practice. They should be read as an introduction. Elsewhere the book is arranged according to topics in alphabetical order, in the format familiar to readers of the series. Cross-reference may be made to other chapters. The chapters on cancer pain are kept together.

We have attempted to organize our topics so that evidence-based medicine is afforded high priority. Yet we accept that much of our practice, and that of those with whom we meet regularly to share clinical problems, is based on precedent and experience. Our sources include comments made by colleagues in lectures at national and international meetings, and informally. It is impossible to acknowledge all of these sources.

The book is dedicated to our trainees and those other professionals who have laboured with us to build up our respective practices. In particular we acknowledge the support of Chris Glynn, Sara Severn, Frank Grady, Alan Severn and Barrie Tait.

*Andrew Severn, Kathryn Grady*

# Names of Medical Substances

In accordance with directive 92/27/EEC, this book adheres to the following guidelines on naming of medicinal substances (rINN, Recommended International Non-proprietary Name; BAN, British Approved Name).

## List 1 – Both names to appear

| UK Name | rINN |
|---|---|
| [1]adrenaline | epinephrine |
| amethocaine | tetracaine |
| bendrofluazide | bendroflumethiazide |
| benzhexol | trihexyphenidyl |
| chlorpheniramine | chlorphenamine |
| dicyclomine | dicycloverine |
| dothiepin | dosulepin |
| eformoterol | formoterol |
| flurandrenolone | fludroxycortide |
| frusemide | furosemide |
| hydroxyurea | hydroxycarbamide |
| lignocaine | lidocaine |
| methotrimeprazine | levomepromazine |
| methylene blue | methylthioninium chloride |
| mitozantrone | mitoxantrone |
| mustine | chlormethine |
| nicoumalone | acenocoumarol |
| [1]noradrenaline | norepinephrine |
| oxypentifylline | pentoxyifylline |
| procaine penicillin | procaine benzylpenicillin |
| salcatonin | calcitonin (salmon) |
| thymoxamine | moxisylyte |
| thyroxine sodium | levothyroxine sodium |
| trimeprazine | alimemazine |

## List 2 – rINN to appear exclusively

| Former BAN | rINN/new BAN |
|---|---|
| amoxycillin | amoxicillin |
| amphetamine | amfetamine |
| amylobarbitone | amobarbital |
| amylobarbitone sodium | amobarbital sodium |

| | |
|---|---|
| beclomethasone | beclometasone |
| benorylate | benorilate |
| busulphan | busulfan |
| butobarbitone | butobarbital |
| carticaine | articane |
| cephalexin | cefalexin |
| cephamandole nafate | cefamandole nafate |
| cephazolin | cefazolin |
| cephradine | cefradine |
| chloral betaine | cloral betaine |
| chlorbutol | chlorobutanol |
| chlormethiazole | clomethiazole |
| chlorathalidone | chlortalidone |
| cholecalciferol | colecalciferol |
| cholestyramine | colestyramine |
| clomiphene | clomifene |
| colistin sulphomethate sodium | colistimethate sodium |
| corticotrophin | corticotropin |
| cysteamine | mercaptamine |
| danthron | dantron |
| desoxymethasone | desoximetasone |
| dexamphetamine | dexamfetamine |
| dibromopropamidine | dibrompropamidine |
| dienoestrol | dienestrol |
| dimethicone(s) | dimeticone |
| dimethyl sulphoxide | dimethyl sulfoxide |
| doxycycline hydrochloride (hemihydrate hemiethanolate) | doxycycline hyclate |
| ethancrynic acid | etacrynic acid |
| ethamsylate | etamsylate |
| ethinyloestradiol | ethinylestradiol |
| ethynodiol | etynodiol |
| flumethasone | flumetasone |
| flupenthixol | flupentixol |
| gestronol | gestonorone |
| guaiphenesin | guaifenesin |

[1] In common with the BP, precedence will continue to be given to the terms adrenaline and noradrenaline.

| | | | |
|---|---|---|---|
| hexachlorophane | hexachlorophene | quinalbarbitone | secobarbital |
| hexamine hippurate | methenamine hippurate | riboflavine | riboflavin |
| | | sodium calciumedetate | sodium calcium edetate |
| hydroxyprogesterone hexanoate | hydroxyprogesterone caproate | sodium cromoglycate | sodium cromoglicate |
| indomethacin | indometacin | sodium ironedetate | sodium feredetate |
| lysuride | lisuride | sodium picosulphate | sodium picosulfate |
| methyl cysteine | mecysteine | sorbitan monostearate | sorbitan stearate |
| methylphenobarbitone | methylphenobarbital | stilboestrol | diethylstilbestrol |
| oestradiol | estradiol | sulphacetamide | sulfacetamide |
| oestriol | estriol | sulphadiazine | sulfadiazine |
| oestrone | estrone | sulphadimidine | sulfadimidine |
| oxethazaine | oxetacaine | sulphaguanadine | sulfaguanadine |
| pentaerythritol tetranitrate | pentaerithrityl tetranitrate | sulphamethoxazole | sulfamethoxazole |
| | | sulphasalazine | sulfasalazine |
| phenobarbitone | phenobarbital | sulphathiazole | sulfathiazole |
| pipothiazine | pipotiazine | sulphinpyrazone | sulfinpyrazone |
| polyhexanide | polihexanide | tetracosactrin | tetracosactide |
| potassium cloazepate | dipotassium clorazepate | thiabendazole | tiabendazole |
| | | thioguanine | tioguanine |
| pramoxine | pramocaine | thiopentone | thiopental |
| prothionamide | protionamide | urofollitrophin | urofollitropin |

# INTRODUCTION – WHAT IS THE PAIN CLINIC?

*Andrew Severn, Kate Grady*

## Scope of the pain clinic

Chronic pain patients are a diverse group of patients, and there is no one recognized medical specialty that can truly claim the responsibility for managing pain. Historically the major impetus for the establishment of specialist pain clinics was cancer pain and the development of techniques for nerve destruction. However, improvement in medical management and nursing care of cancer patients has in most cases superseded the need for techniques that prompted such specialist interest. The focus of attention of many pain clinics has thus become one of managing a condition that is usefully called a chronic pain syndrome, rather than the symptomatic treatment of pain symptoms. The general hospital pain clinic manages cancer pain, nerve injury pain, chronic back problems and peripheral vascular disease. Its involvement may be for technical service reasons, such as a sympathectomy to improve blood flow to the ischaemic limb, or it may take the lead role in managing the complex medical and psychosocial problem called the chronic pain syndrome.

The Royal College of Anaesthetists recognizes the specialty of 'pain management' and is responsible for the training of anaesthesia specialists and the recognition of consultant anaesthetist posts. The Pain Society, affiliated to the Association of Anaesthetists of Great Britain and Ireland is the UK chapter of the International Association for the Study of Pain (IASP). The membership of the Pain Society and IASP is interdisciplinary.

## Pain as a disease

The chronic pain syndrome is the end result of a variety of pathological and psychological mechanisms that may have included, at some stage, tissue or nerve damage, and in which symptoms have failed to resolve with healing or repair. It is helpful to consider the chronic pain syndrome as a disease in its own right. Chronic pain syndrome has its own symptomatology, signs and natural history that can be recognized in many patients irrespective of the primary source of the symptoms of pain. The management of the chronic pain syndrome requires the clinician to shift emphasis from the relief of the pain to the prevention of complications and the rehabilitation of the sufferer, a role similar to that of a physician managing any other chronic condition. Symptomatic relief is of less importance than the development of a strategy for long-term management. While it is noted that short-term relief of pain symptoms is reported with many techniques, both 'conventional' and 'complementary', the prospects of these interventions to deliver long-lasting changes in function and behaviour is by no means as certain. Indeed, there are risks of any technique that provides short-term relief but does not address the consequences of chronic pain, namely that the sufferer relies on the professional for repeated intervention. In practice this means that establishment of a service providing a low-cost, minimally invasive modality of treatment, for example, using acupuncture, commits the clinician to a long-term, open-ended relationship with the patient unless some form of 'contract' is agreed with the patient. Agreement has to be made with patient and health care purchaser that sees a course of treatment designed not only to provide symptomatic relief but also to reduce disability and encourage a return to normal activity. One way of assessing the effectiveness of treatment is to shift the line of enquiry from 'did it hurt less?' to 'did you manage to do more?'. It is important that the patient understands this role. The patient needs to be aware of his or her own responsibility to maintain any gains which have been achieved in the pain clinic.

The contract between pain clinic and the purchaser of the service must therefore reflect the type and extent of rehabilitation work that needs to be undertaken by the pain clinic. Two features that have to be addressed are the length of time for which follow up is necessary and the number and role of other professions that need to be formally involved. The growth in number and variety of interested professionals means that there is no one model of care provision that needs to be accepted as 'standard'. Without standardization it is difficult to decide on an outcome that allows the patient to be returned from the supervision of the clinic to the supervision of the primary care team. Desired outcomes will vary, depending on the type of referral and the ability of primary care to take on responsibility for long-term monitoring. It is to be expected that there will be frequent requests for review of the pain symptoms and advice on management of the condition of chronic pain.

### Relationship with other medical bodies

Investigation of ongoing pathology is not the role of the clinic, although a working knowledge of screening for and referral of suspected rheumatological and neurological disease is required. This is best obtained by discussion with local specialists. Similarly, local negotiation will define the limits of responsibility for the management of conditions such as headache, back pain, osteoporosis and cancer. In general terms, attendance at the pain clinic assumes that all reasonable attempts at diagnosis and management of ongoing disease have been addressed by relevant specialists. Some acceptance of the unique role of the clinic as a resource for the management of a chronic condition is however desirable. It may be convenient for a pain clinic to take on the major role for symptom relief from other specialists, for example for the performing of procedures such as epidural injections, but the wider need for rehabilitation in this group of patients must not be lost in the press of referrals for interventions with only short-term proven benefit.

### Clinical governance

Clinical governance is a doctrine that the clinician is responsible to the employing authority, as well as his professional body, for aspects of professional conduct. The pain clinician may therefore expect to be involved in advising the employer about issues concerning the management of patients under the care of colleagues, and in advising about policies that may affect many patients. Conversely, it is important that where clinical experience dictates the use of an approach or techniques for which high-level evidence is unavailable or unconvincing, appropriate measures are taken to ensure that clinical and management colleagues are aware of the clinical reasoning. Prescribing outside a manufacturer's product licence is a case in point. In this case it may be valuable that the employer endorses the practice after consideration by a Drugs and Therapeutics Committee or similar. The consultant has a special responsibility for monitoring the patient on unlicensed medication that may be difficult to delegate to primary care or a trainee.

Pain clinics treat patients who may have failed to respond to conventional medical treatments carried out by other specialists. Some of them have complaints about the way in which they have been treated, others about the complications of which they believe that were not warned. Although the complaint itself may require investigation and an appropriate answer, the process of complaining may be part of the presentation of the disease. The employer therefore has to be prepared to recognize that over-solicitous apology for an alleged inaction may reinforce the behaviour and lead to repeated frustrations and complaints.

## Relationship with non-medical bodies

The clinician is encouraged to extend influence beyond the immediate medical community to the self-help groups that meet outside hospitals. Many of them understand the strategy of management of chronic pain. Some do not, and may have as their *raison d'être* a commitment to see the provision of a service which is at odds with the clinician's professional judgement. The influence of such groups may be considerable, particularly when they are well organized, skilfully administered, registered as charities, and have the support of well known personalities. These groups have more information available to them through the Internet, and may have access through this medium to 'specialists' whose views may be very different from the local clinic. The clinician is advised not to ignore the local impact and support that these groups often have, even if some conflict is involved. It is well worth finding out what groups exist, what access there is to information on the Internet and where the agenda of the group differs from that of the clinician. Common grounds for mutual support may be found, even when there is disagreement about some aspects of the aims of the group. Similarly, such groups may be considered allies in the quest for resources, although the clinician must keep the aims of the group subject to his professional judgement when deciding what types of treatment should be provided with such resources.

## Medicolegal reporting

The role of the legal system is to decide what is genuine and to compensate appropriately where there is blame. The area of chronic pain presents problems in trying to do this. For those without understanding of pain and its mechanisms the concept of pain following injury that does not resolve after tissue healing is difficult to grasp. Further difficulty arises because chronic pain is often reported where there is no obvious pathology. Moreover chronic pain in itself manifests a variety of psychological features and behavioural adaptations or 'inconsistencies' which may be perceived as fraudulent or malingering behaviour. At the centre of the legal problem is the question 'Is the patient attempting to deceive or exaggerate?' There is no precise way to know. However although the report of pain may be said to be entirely subjective, for those with specialist knowledge there may be features in the history which give objectivity as they are spontaneous reports of what the patient would be unlikely to know e.g. 'it's numb but it hurts' or on examination, the demonstration of allodynia. It remains however that there are pains for which there is no objective evidence and this group will always be questioned as genuine.

The very specialized duty of the pain clinician to the court in medicolegal reporting of chronic pain cases is to provide assessment of presence and degree of pain by the professional interpretation of history and signs on examination, to provide explanation as to why a pain may be ongoing, and to describe the 'normal' features of a chronic pain syndrome. Illness behaviour can be thought of as an expression that the patient is suffering pain.

## Outpatient procedures

Nerve block of a major nerve trunk requires facilities for resuscitation and monitoring, together with an aseptic environment. Such procedures are optimally undertaken in a day case operating theatre. X-ray imaging facilities are required for precise localization in many procedures. This can usually be achieved with biplanar screening with a C-arm intensifier that can rotate around the patient. Computed tomography is valuable for some procedures, such as coeliac plexus block. Sedation and general anaesthesia requires a comprehensive facility for monitoring, recovery, and of appropriately trained personnel to supervise the patient while the clinician undertakes the procedure. Very minor procedures, such as trigger point injection or greater occipital nerve block can be undertaken in the outpatient clinic.

# ASSESSMENT OF EVIDENCE – EVIDENCE IN DECISION-MAKING

*Andrew Smith*

## Bias

Bias is the term we give to something which hinders us from getting a true picture, whether it is in a television news report, an opinion poll or scientific research. As clinicians we need unbiased information, and one of the benefits of the evidence-based medicine 'movement' is that it has encouraged us to look for reliable, valid, unbiased sources of evidence to inform our clinical practice. It also promotes the idea that we should all be capable of evaluating what we read and detecting bias for ourselves. These chapters are designed to give a simple guide to sources of bias in clinical evidence and how they can be overcome.

First let us look at a simple fictitious example. A medical electronics company is marketing a new radiofrequency lesion generator. Is it any good?

Often clinicians' responses to that question include the following:

- 'I don't know but I liked the colour of the casing and the controls were easy to use'.
- 'I don't know but the company rep paid for me to go to an international meeting last year so I thought I'd better try it'.
- 'Professor X said it was good at the Pain Society meeting last month'.
- 'I'm going to suggest it to Mrs Y at her next clinic visit as I've tried almost everything else'.
- 'I used it on a patient last week and it worked a treat'.
- 'I used it on a patient last week and she's no better'.

Now, leaving aside the distinctly non-clinical issues of equipment design and relationships between doctors and medical manufacturers, these responses throw up some interesting points about evidence. The doctor who quotes Professor X suggests that his expert authority (even though it is based on the Professor's own experience as no formal evaluation has yet been performed) is in some way better than his own assessment. Mrs Y's doctor wants the new generator to work as she needs help. This is only natural but already he is biased in its favour and cannot be said to be approaching it with an open mind. The two doctors who have tried it – on one patient each – have both made up their minds about it but have come to different conclusions. So who is right? Does the new generator work?

Of course the right answer is that nobody knows – yet. It is time for independent properly conducted clinical trials of the new device comparing it with the best available existing device. Only when we have that sort of evidence will we be able to start setting the new machine in its rightful clinical context. But how often is such evidence available?

## Levels of evidence

The idea of a hierarchy of evidence is now quite well known. A typical example is shown as Table 1. If you have to make a treatment decision, you should choose a therapy whose effectiveness has been demonstrated by a well-conducted systematic review (see *Reviews: traditional and modern*). Failing that, it should be supported by a sound randomized controlled trial (RCT). Beyond that, the evidence from the different types of study is thought to be less and less robust as you move down the order. Although typical hierarchies have only these five categories, clinicians have always operated on evidence, but often based on personal experience ('I had a patient once who . . .') or that of others ('Dr X had a patient once who . . .'). This may be only human but is not thought to be as reliable as the higher levels.

**Table 1.** Typical hierarchy of evidence

| | |
|---|---|
| I | Systematic review of RCTs |
| II | Single RCT |
| III | Observational studies e.g. cohort studies |
| IV | Case series |
| V | Case report |

Whilst it remains true that the RCT, and hence, quantitative meta-analyses derived from RCTs, provide the best available current evidence for effectiveness of therapies, they are not the best way of answering every question arising from our clinical practice. For instance, many RCTs do not examine adverse effects of treatments, and these can be important in determining patient compliance. Case reports do not provide a powerful basis for the effectiveness of a treatment, but can be very useful for publicizing complications such as adverse drug reactions. Nonetheless, the RCT has achieved 'cultural supremacy' amongst clinical research methods so it is examined in more detail below.

## The randomized controlled trial

The randomized controlled trial (RCT) has been used in medicine since the 1940s. Improvements in methodology mean that, for appropriate research questions, results can be obtained with a very low risk of bias.

As time has passed, the methodological rigour of clinical investigations has increased. Whereas at one time, uncontrolled observational studies of new treatments were the norm, now random allocation into one or more groups is standard.

Some element of blinding, that is, hiding from patients, their doctors and sometimes others, which group patients are in, is usual. These two steps – allocation concealment and blinding – are thought to be the two most important in reducing bias.

Non-randomized studies tend to overestimate the effects of new treatments when compared with placebo. However, our understanding of the potentials and limitations of the RCT has advanced, and it is now clear that a number of potential biaises can operate. These are outlined below.

**1. Participation bias.** Simply taking part in a clinical trial can distort the behaviour of clinicians and their patients. Usually this is neither deliberate nor fraudulent. The fact remains that patients in the control groups of RCTs tend to fare better than patients on identical treatments (whether it be placebo or the best available current treatment) who are not being studied. This may be due to more intensive monitoring and greater attention from clinicians, or may result from selection bias (see below).

**2. Selection bias.** Ethical probity demands that patients have to be informed about the risks and benefits of participation in the trial and give their formal consent to taking part. Although right and proper, this introduces another potential bias. Not all patients approached will agree to take part, and this has two consequences. First, patients who take part in trials may be different in some way from those who do not. Hence, whilst the results of the trial may hold true for the patients studied, they may not be more widely applicable. In particular, it may be one reason why it can be difficult to reproduce the findings of a trial in clinical practice. Second, however, one can get a measure of how acceptable the intervention sounds to patients. If only a small proportion of those approached actually agree to take part, it may be that the intervention is rather unpleasant. Although these figures are often not reported, they can give useful information on acceptability.

**3. Allocation bias.** The greatest benefit of randomization is that it controls not only for known confounding factors, but also for unknown ones. True randomization should be distinguished from what are often called 'quasi-random' methods of allocation such as using the last digit of the patient's hospital number (odd/even) or the referring clinician. While these might seem innocuous at first sight, they can hide potentially important differences. For instance, a pain specialist whose clinics are held on a Tuesday might have more complex cases than one who consults on a Wednesday, thus introducing baseline differences right from the start. Currently, the most robust method of allocation concealment is thought to be using random number tables to produce cards which are then sealed in opaque envelopes to be opened when a patient is to be allocated a group.

**4. Performance, observation and analysis bias.** If patients know which group they are in, their perception of their health may be altered: for instance, if they know they have been given a new 'wonder drug' they may be more likely to report benefit. Clinicians too are only human and even when they are trying to be impartial may convey certain expectations to patients through their manner or choice of words. The term *double-blind* is applied when neither the patient, nor the person treating them, knows which group the patient is in. However, this does not guarantee an unbiased outcome. If someone else again is assessing the effect of the intervention, they should also be blinded to the groups. Ideally, those who are analysing the results should be blinded too. Strictly speaking, such a trial would then be *quadruple blind*!

**5. Inference bias and the role of peer review.** Inference bias refers to the tendency of some researchers to draw conclusions from their research when these are not justified from the data themselves. It is thus not uncommon for a trial to show, for example, a 20% reduction in average pain scores with a new analgesic, but to draw the conclusion 'all patients should receive this agent as first-line treatment' is another matter altogether. There is nothing wrong with opinion in itself. Difficulties arise, however, when opinion is presented as evidence. In a way one can say that research findings only really exist once they have been published – they are likely to influence only a small number of people until they appear in print. Because of this, the editorial process of scientific journals may influence the dissemination of research. Papers are reviewed by one or more experts, whose advice on publication may lead to rejection.

## What do we do when there is no evidence?

Having levels of evidence in our minds, as they are throughout this book, is all very well and good, but what if the patient presents with a condition for which there is no good evidence from systematic reviews or RCTs? What if there are only two RCTs or two systematic reviews and their conclusions disagree? In this case, it is possible to go through the original trials or reviews to see if the point of divergence can be identified, but sometimes there is genuine uncertainty about an intervention. So-called lesser levels of evidence may then have to suffice, and if this constitutes the best available evidence then that is all we can hope for – until something better comes along. But what if there really is no evidence? The first point to remember is that lack of evidence does not simply mean lack of benefit. Public health specialists and policy-makers are often keen to take the view that if an intervention has not been shown to be effective, then it should not be funded. This is somewhat extreme. But the question is not just a philosophical and ethical one. All interventions carry benefits and risks. If we are using an unevaluated, unproven intervention which has not been shown to be beneficial, then we are putting patients at risk of harm without offering them any benefit. Should we continue to use that intervention? On the other hand, it is possible that the treatment is indeed beneficial, in which case we will deny patients that benefit if we stop using it. Such uncertainty over the net effects of a treatment should prompt us to do two things. First, it should trigger a search for such evidence as there may be about the treatment. Second, if there isn't any, we should try to establish some. If sufficient uncertainty exists as to which of a number of interventions is best – so-called clinical equipoise – then this is the perfect opportunity for a randomized controlled trial.

Patients and their doctors like to have clear-cut answers to questions about diagnosis, treatment and prognosis. However, we cannot always make unequivocal statements about effectiveness.

When there isn't any evidence (see *bias and levels of evidence*) we are thrown back on our clinical judgement and compassion. Even when evidence is present, patients do not always welcome it. For many, the accumulated experience of a seasoned clinician is enough. And, worse, what if no effective treatment is available – when there is 'nothing more we can do'? Although Archie Cochrane's name is now firmly associated with evidence-based medicine, he knew only too well, as medical officer in a prisoner-of-war camp in World War II, the importance of common kindness and humanity, as this extract from his autobiography, in which he attends to a dying Russian soldier, shows:

'... The ward was full, so I put him in my room as he was moribund and screaming and I did not want to wake the ward. I examined him. He had obvious gross bilateral cavitation and a severe pleural rub. I thought the latter was the cause of the pain and screaming. I had no morphia, just aspirin, which had no effect. I felt desperate. I knew very little Russian then and there was no one in the ward who did. I finally instinctively sat down on the bed and took him in my arms, and the screaming stopped almost at once. He died peacefully in my arms a few hours later. It was not the pleurisy that caused the screaming, but loneliness. It was a wonderful education about the care of the dying.' (From Cochrane AL *One Man's Medicine: The Autobiography of Archie Cochrane*. London: BMJ Memoir Club, 1988. Reproduced with permission.)

## Further reading

Jadad AR. *Randomised Controlled Trials*. London: BMJ Books, 1998.
Vandenbroucke JP. Case reports in an evidence-based world. *Journal of the Royal Society of Medicine*, 1999; **92:** 159–63.

# ASSESSMENT OF EVIDENCE – EVIDENCE-BASED MEDICINE AND THE SCIENCE OF REVIEWING RESEARCH

*Andrew Smith*

## Evidence-based medicine

The idea of evidence-based medicine (EBM) arose from the writings of the Scottish epidemiologist Archie Cochrane, most famously his book *Effectiveness and Efficiency*, first published in 1972. These were taken up and publicized by David Sackett and colleagues at McMaster University in Canada in the late 1970s and 1980s. Cochrane argued that much of medical practice was not based on good scientific evidence, and suggested that the randomized controlled trial be used more widely to show which interventions were beneficial and which not.

There are five simple steps:

1. *Ask a clinical question you can answer.* A good question specifies intervention, subjects and outcome.
2. *Search for evidence.* Usually on computerized databases such as Medline.
3. *Critically appraise the evidence.* Is the research of good quality? Are the results important and useful for me as a clinician?
4. *Integrate the evidence into practice.* Decide how (or if) it applies to the patient.
5. *Evaluate the process.* Did it work? Could we have done it better?

Now the idea of going back to primary sources of research to answer clinical questions is not new. What is novel, however, is the exhortation that ordinary doctors and other healthcare workers should do it for themselves rather than rely on others. This brings with it great potential benefits.

Evidence-based medicine offers at once a way of making the medical literature more manageable, a way of answering problems arising in clinical practice, a way of keeping up to date and a way of finding what helps patients and what does not. It offers a vision of a utopian medical world where healthcare workers act to bring about the greatest good for the greatest number as they apply the fruits of their own expert appraisal of the scientific basis of healthcare.

In reality, there are a number of problems. The practice of evidence-based medicine as described above needs skills which most doctors, nurses and therapists simply do not have. Searching can be, and is often best done, by a trained medical librarian, and applying the results in practice is seldom a problem for practising clinicians. It is the process of critical appraisal that causes difficulty. Research methodology is developing rapidly in itself and to understand the nuances of method can be challenging. Nonetheless, the basic principles are straightforward and the widely held view that interpreting research needs a detailed knowledge of biostatistics is not true. Poor-quality papers are usually poor because the authors have asked the wrong question, or gone about answering it in the wrong way, or lost the logical thread of argument in the discussion.

Also, the practice of evidence-based medicine clearly takes up considerable time, and consequently it is unusual for busy clinicians to go through the steps above for more than a handful of clinical problems. We need summaries and we need others to interpret the literature for us. These sources are potentially very useful but readers need to keep their wits about them when using them too (see *Review articles: traditional and modern*). The idea of evidence-based medicine is illusory in that it implies that every clinical problem can be answered. This is clearly not true and raises practical as well as philosophical problems (see *Evidence: what to do when there isn't any*). Nonetheless, if the evidence-based medicine movement does nothing else, it will have achieved something worthwhile if it stimulates those who use medical scientific information to adopt a critical attitude to published evidence and expert pronouncements. The answer to any question should always be followed by another, namely 'And where's the evidence for that?'.

## Evidence: reviews, traditional and modern

Review articles have always been popular with busy doctors as they offer an up-to-date summary of published work on a topic of interest. In 1987 Mulrow, in a widely-cited paper, alleged that traditional review articles – where an expert selects what he considers relevant and then adds his own opinion – is subjective and prone to bias. This may not necessarily be true but it is often not clear what is fact and what is opinion and ideally readers should be able to distinguish the two and make up their own minds. The systematic review is put forward as a solution to this problem. A systematic review has a clearly defined protocol governing how carefully papers are sought, how decisions about inclusion/exclusion are made, how the quality of the various papers affects their validity, and how the results of different papers are combined into a conclusion. By making the review process visible, the reader is allowed to judge its quality – and hence the validity of its conclusions and recommendations – in a way which is impossible in the older type of review.

Essentially a systematic review is a pre-planned investigation in itself. If one were planning a clinical trial, one would set out in advance, in the form of a protocol, what the research question was, who would be studied, how the results would be analysed and so on. The systematic review uses the same principles. The term *secondary research* is often used to describe the science of systematic reviews, to contrast it with the primary studies on which the reviews are based. This is useful because it connotes a more methodical approach, but also because it implies by association that biases can creep in here, just as they can into RCTs.

Systematic reviews can be prone to a number of biases, which can potentially affect the review's validity and usefulness.

*1. Selection bias.* Arises from inadequate searching – some RCTs are missed. This could alter the results.

*2. Publication and language bias.* It is known that some studies are more likely to be published than others. For instance, those with positive findings are more likely to get into print than those with negative findings, though both may be equally valid. Likewise, Medline, being a North American database, is biased towards material published in English. Searches should not be limited by language as the English-speaking world does not have a monopoly on sound research.

**3.** *Inclusion and appraisal bias.* The process by which studies are judged suitable or unsuitable for inclusion should be clearly laid out. Sometimes it can be difficult to decide, but this should be made explicit and the reasons for a particular choice given. Appraisal refers to the process of judging the soundness of the study. Although quality checklists for assessing RCTs are available, different individuals may disagree about the strengths and weaknesses of a study. Ideally, more than one person should make decisions about inclusion and quality and sources of disagreement explored and laid bare.

**4.** *Inference and reviewer bias.* The temptation for reviewers to make unjustified leaps from data to conclusion is still present just as for RCTs. Peer reviewers of the review, too, may allow their personal biases to influence the final shape of the work.
Template for a systematic review:

1. Decide scope and purpose (the first step for evidence-based medicine, 'ask a clear clinical question' is a good guide here too). This is a critical stage as too wide a scope could make for an unmanageable amount of data. The other issue to resolve is whether to review subjects where there is a lot of published material ('data-driven') even when the subject is not a burning issue, or choose a topic to which we really need an answer even though there may not be many data to inform it ('question driven').
2. Perform an exhaustive search for material. A quick Medline search is only the starting point, and systematic reviewers often search other databases, specialized registers of trials and hand-search journals likely to contain material on the chosen topic. The risk is that the studies which are easier to find are somehow different from the others. Unless one can locate all the relevant material, the review's conclusions could be biased. Unpublished studies can be especially hard to find – conference abstracts and direct contact with researchers in the topic area can be helpful.
3. Include or exclude studies on pre-defined criteria. Usually randomization is the first and most important criterion, but other methodological aspects and outcome measures may influence this.
4. Extract data. Sometimes, the data as reported in the article are not sufficient to establish what happened in the RCT, or are presented in a format which cannot be compared with other RCTs. In these cases, contacting the authors directly can help.
5. Perform quality assessment of included studies. This relates mostly to allocation concealment and blinding as they have the greatest influence on validity.
6. Synthesis and integration. Often, the statistical techniques of meta-analysis are applied to give a numerical estimate of combined treatment effect. This is not always possible, for instance when the primary studies are too dissimilar, but allows the calculation of odd ratios, numbers needed to treat (NNTs) etc. (see *Expressing and Interpreting the Results of Research*).
7. Interpretation. It is only right that reviewers should have the chance to comment on what they have found. Being involved in a systematic review allows you to explore a subject in great depth and gives you a perspective on it which cannot be fully expressed in a 'bottom-line' odds ratio. It should be made clear, however, that this is opinion and not part of the evidence base.

Reviewers' conclusions on the data are specifically labelled as such in reviews within the Cochrane Collaboration and this is to be welcomed. For instance, statements such as 'All patients with condition X should receive treatment Y' should not appear. That should be for the clinician looking after the patient to decide.

Note that, simply because a review is labelled systematic, it is not necessarily better than a traditional narrative review. The parallels with primary research continue in that, just as adopting the RCT format does not absolve researchers from the responsibility of having to think about what they are doing, so using the systematic review format does not in itself provide high-quality evidence. As always, readers ideally need to be able to judge for themselves, and the benefit of the systematic approach is that it makes the review process more transparent and allows the reader to see how the conclusions were reached.

## Evidence: the Cochrane Collaboration

In 1979, Archie Cochrane (see *Evidence-Based Medicine*) challenged the medical profession to put together, by specialty, a critical summary of randomized controlled trials to enable medical practice to be put on a sounder footing of evidence. Rightly or wrongly, he singled out obstetrics as that branch of healthcare most in need of this approach. Iain Chalmers and others took up this challenge, and the result was the book *Effective Care in Pregnancy and Childbirth*. Such was the book's success that it was later released on floppy disk as the *Oxford Database of Perinatal Trials*. This systematic approach to collating research evidence found favour within the UK National Health Service Research and Development Programme of 1991, and the world's first Cochrane Centre was opened in Oxford in 1992, with Iain Chalmers as its first director. The Cochrane Collaboration evolved from this and is now a worldwide venture whose aims are to prepare, maintain and disseminate systematic reviews (see *Reviews: traditional and modern*) of the effects of healthcare interventions.

There are now 14 Cochrane Centres all over the world, co-ordinating a growing number of review groups. The Collaboration publishes the *Cochrane Library*, which contains over 1000 completed Cochrane systematic reviews, the Database of Abstracts of Reviews of Effectiveness (high-quality reviews from non-Cochrane sources), and the Controlled Clinical Trials Register, with over 294 000 clinical trials. The *Library* is updated every 3 months on CD-ROM and is also available on line.

Individuals wishing to undertake a review contact the Review Group covering their proposed subject. The Review Group Co-ordinator checks that the subject is not already being reviewed and, if not, registers the review title. The reviewers then prepare a protocol setting out their search strategy, inclusion criteria and other aspects of method. When approved by peer reviewers and the Group's editorial team, the protocol is published on the Cochrane Library. The Group then supports the reviewers throughout the review process and the finished review is also published, again after satisfactory internal and external scrutiny. An important part of the reviewers' task is to update the review periodically as new material becomes available. The electronic format of the Library makes this technically straight-forward.

Further information can be found at **www.cochrane.org** and abstracts can be viewed at http//hiru.mcmaster.ca/cochrane/cochrane/cdsr/htm

Most areas of healthcare are now represented and reviews dealing with chronic pain have found their way onto the Library through various Review Groups – for instance, the Musculoskeletal Group maintains the reviews on interventions for low back pain. There is, however, a Cochrane Pain, Palliative and Supportive Care Group. The Group has 13 completed reviews and 17 protocols published on Issue 2, 2001 of the Cochrane Library.

Reviews include:

- Acupuncture for idiopathic headache.
- Anticonvulsant drugs for acute and chronic pain.
- Radiotherapy for the palliation of painful bone metastases.
- Surgery for the resolution of symptoms in malignant bowel obstruction in advanced gynaecological and gastrointestinal cancer.

Protocols include:

- Bisphosphonates as analgesics for pain secondary to bone metastases.
- Noninvasive physical treatments for chronic headache.
- Opioids for the palliation of breathlessness in terminal illness.

The group is based in Oxford and correspondence should be addressed to:
Frances Fairman
Review Group Co-ordinator
Pain Relief Unit
Churchill Hospital
Oxford OX3 7LJ (UK)

E-mail: frances.fairman@pru.ox.ac.uk
www.jr2.ox.ac.uk/cochrane

## Further reading

Egger M, Davey Smith G, Altman D, eds. *Systematic Reviews in Health Care*, 2nd Edn. London: British Medical Journal Books, 2001.

Greenhalgh T. *How to read a paper*, 2nd Edn. London: British Medical Journal Books, 2000.

Petticrew M. Systematic reviews from astronomy to zoology: Myths and Misconceptions. British Medical Journal, 2001; **322:** 98–101.

Sackett DL *et al. Evidence-based medicine. How to practise and teach EBM*. Edinburgh: Churchill Livingstone, 1997.

# ASSESSMENT OF EVIDENCE –
# EXPRESSING AND INTERPRETING
# THE RESULTS OF RESEARCH

*Andrew Smith*

This example uses a fictitious randomized controlled trial of a new anticonvulsant, gabatryptiline, for the treatment of neuropathic pain. In all, 1092 patients take part, of whom 529 receive the active treatment and 563 the control drug. The outcome in question is a 50% reduction in severity of pain. Of the patients taking gabatryptiline, 378 responded as opposed to 303 of those taking the control drug.

Expressing these results in a two by two table, we get:

|          | Responded | Did not respond | Total |
|----------|-----------|-----------------|-------|
| Active   | 378       | 151             | 529   |
| Control  | 303       | 260             | 563   |
| Total    | 681       | 411             | 1092  |

The **risk** (or probability) of having pain in the gabatryptiline group is 151/529 which is 0.29.

The **baseline risk** of having pain (control group) is 260/563 which is 0.46.

The **risk ratio** (or **relative risk**) is the gabatryptiline risk divided by the baseline risk, that is 0.29/0.46 which works out at 0.63.

The **odds** of having pain in the gabatryptiline group are 151/378 which is 0.4.

The **baseline odds** of having pain are 260/303 which is 0.86.

The **odds ratio** is the gabatryptiline odds divided by the baseline odds, that is 0.4/0.86 which works out at 0.46.

If the outcome in question is rare, the risk ratio and the odds ratio are numerically similar. As the observed outcome becomes more frequent (as it is in this example) then their values diverge.

The **absolute risk reduction** is calculated by subtracting the gabatryptiline risk from the baseline risk, that is 0.46−0.29, which is 0.17 or 17%.

The **relative risk reduction** is calculated by subtracting the gabatryptiline risk from the baseline risk and dividing by the baseline risk, that is (0.46−0.29)/0.46. This works out at 0.37 or 37%.

The **number needed to treat** (NNT) tells us how many patients need to be treated with gabatryptiline for one to benefit. It is simply the reciprocal of the absolute risk reduction, or 1/0.17, which works out at 6.

An analogous measure is the **number needed to harm** (NNH). Although, as often happens in clinical trials of new agents, no attempt has been made to quantify adverse effects, this gives a measure of how commonly patients experience side effects. For instance, a NNH of 5 for drowsiness means that, on average, one patient will feel drowsy for every 5 patients taking the drug.

So the same results from the same trial can be expressed in a number of different ways. It has been shown that doctors, patients and policymakers do not always understand the significance of these different formats. The relative risk reduction of 37%, for instance, sounds much more impressive, and is likely to sell more gabatryptiline, than an absolute risk reduction of 17%, but they mean the same. However, they both convey more than the odds ratio to the uninitiated reader. The number needed to treat, on the other hand, has become popular because it combines an easily understood concept with the level-headed sobriety of the absolute risk reduction. It also allows a comparison of different drugs even though they may not have been compared directly in the same clinical study. Numbers needed to treat have been calculated for a number of analgesics in acute pain and have allowed the construction of a 'league table'. For instance, paracetamol 1 g with codeine 60 mg is at the top of the table, with a NNT of 2 (to achieve 50% pain relief) whereas tramadol 75 mg, with a NNT of 5, cannot be recommended so strongly.

The way potential benefits and risks are communicated to patients can influence their decision whether or not to accept the treatment. Leaving aside the issue of which of the above ways one chooses to use, other factors can also play their part. For instance, patients may be more likely to start, and persevere with, a treatment that is presented as giving them a 30% chance of feeling better rather than as one with a 70% chance of feeling the same. This is known as 'positive framing' and is only one of many influences reviewed by Bogardus and colleagues in their review.

## Further reading

Analgesic league tables can be viewed at: www.jr2.ox.ac.uk/Bandolier/painres/painpag/Acutrev/Analgesics/Leaguetab.html

Bogardus ST, Holmboe E, Jekel JF. Perils, pitfalls and possibilities in talking about medical risk. *Journal of the American Medical Association*, 1999; **281**: 1037–41.

Greenhalgh T. *How to read a paper.* London: BMJ Books, 2nd ed., 2000.

Sterne JAC, Davey Smith G. Sifting the evidence – what's wrong with significance tests? *British Medical Journal*, 2001; **322**: 226–31.

# ASSESSMENT OF CHRONIC PAIN – HISTORY

*Kate Grady, Andrew Severn*

It is helpful to consider chronic pain as a disease in which many factors, physical, pathological and psychosocial contribute to the presentation. Thus the history itself is more than the history of the symptoms which provide diagnostic clues, the traditional model on which medical science is based. The clinician taking a history of chronic pain must be prepared to set aside preconceptions on which traditional medical diagnosis is taught. For example, standard teaching may suggest that pain that is experienced in a 'glove' or 'stocking' distribution is in some way 'fraudulent' because it does not fit with a preconceived anatomical knowledge of the sensory dermatomes. From the perspective of the pain clinic symptoms of pain should be recorded as they are experienced, without prejudice to the clinician's view of the mechanisms involved. Contributing psychosocial factors need to be noted, with the understanding that they are likely to be present, and in a way that the patient is not blamed for the presentation. Most importantly, since the aim of management of chronic pain is a reduction in disability and return of function, the history must include factors such as the impact of the pain on normal functioning. To achieve this the context of history taking is wide: patients, self rating questionnaires, pain diagrams and diaries and the perspective of relatives all offer further information. Discussion of the pain with the patient allows psychological signs to be manifest. Although a diagnosis is less sought after in the pain clinic than in other settings, pathology better managed in other clinics has to be excluded. Traditional medical teaching identifies so-called screening 'red flags' in presentation of illness that mandate the focused search for serious pathology such as cancer or inflammatory disease. Pain clinic history taking uses an analogous screening technique for elements in the psychosocial presentation. We will refer to them as 'yellow flags' to distinguish them from the 'red flags': they are not life-threatening symptoms, but their presence means that the psychosocial history has to be clearly focused. They are symptoms that may need addressing in their own right with psychological treatments.

## The pain

1. **The site** of pain may indicate an underlying local cause, a referred origin, a dermatomal or peripheral nerve distribution or may bear no relationship to traditional neuroanatomical patterns. The site of pain should be recorded as it is reported, without interpretation by the doctor as to the possible diagnosis.

2. **The nature.** Duration, rapidity of onset, whether a pain is intermittent or constant, how it varies in severity with time and circumstance and its overall progression or deterioration determine its nature.

3. **The character** of pain will point to its somatic, visceral or neuropathic component. Descriptions of nociceptive and neuropathic pain can be difficult to distinguish because of significant overlap of symptoms. The description may use words such as 'torturing' or 'cruel', that indicate a level of distress which may need formal evaluation.

**4. *Alleviating and exacerbating*** factors offer information about aetiology. All factors which have a bearing on pain should be considered. Pain that is reported as being relieved by rest may be considered as a 'yellow flag'; pain affected by heat suggests a sympathetic nervous system component.

**5. *The severity*** of pain can be recorded as a numerical categorical scale score. In its simplest form this can be descriptive – the patient is asked, verbally to rate the pain on an arbitrary numerical scale. Visual analogue scales are more sophisticated scoring systems in which the patient marks the score between two points on paper or a simple proprietary model, such as a thermometer.

**6. *The impact*** of pain is assessment of disability and social and personal incapacity caused by pain. It attempts to identify all factors affected by pain. Assessment of impact can contribute to the psychosocial assessment where it reveals personal gain which may result from continuing pain.

## Treatments for pain

Details of all past treatments and their outcomes build a picture of the pain and avoid further futile attempts with the same modalities. However, history should determine whether treatment was effectively prescribed and whether compliance was adequate before considering it a failure. Current treatments and their effects should be noted. The patient may have beliefs about treatment which usefully contribute to psychological assessment, such as their condition being incurable because no treatment has ever worked, an unshakeable belief in a particular treatment and unreasonable expectations from treatments they have not yet tried. These features are 'yellow flags'.

## Other medical history

Other symptoms or conditions can have a bearing on the pain itself or on proposed pain clinic treatments. Current medication for other conditions should be noted, especially where drugs may affect the clinician's willingness to perform a nerve block e.g. anticoagulants.

## Psychosocial history

An understanding of the patient's environment is central to understanding the pain. It assesses logistics of domestic and physical support which would be needed for treatments such as day case procedures, the application of transcutaneous electrical nerve stimulation (TENS) machines and coping with the side-effects of some drugs.

It looks for psychological aspects of the pain. Psychological assessment begins at the first point of contact and does not require the skills of a psychologist initially. Details of personal, sexual and family relationships, source of income, occupation, ethnic origin, availability of social and psychological support can be sought from the history.

The patient's beliefs about the condition and its progression and expectations of treatment should be asked. Beliefs that imply that the patient is seriously worried about the progression of undiagnosed pathology are 'yellow flags'. Symptoms of anxiety, depression or anger are frequently present and may or may not require therapy. A profile of the patient's activities of daily living and questioning about interpersonal relationships demonstrates behavioural components to pain. Outstanding litigation or compensation claims should be recorded.

## Further reading

Bonica JJ. Organization and function of a pain clinic. *Advances in Neurology*, 1974; **4**: 433–43.

## Related topics of interest

Assessment of chronic pain – psychosocial (p. 25); Back pain – medical management (p. 29); Neuropathic pain – an overview (p. 113); Nociceptive pain – an overview (p. 117).

# ASSESSMENT OF
# CHRONIC PAIN – EXAMINATION

*Kate Grady, Paul Eldridge*

This chapter addresses the basics of physical assessment. In other areas of medicine, the physical examination helps to form a diagnosis. In chronic pain the physical assessment has several purposes.

## Purpose

*1.    To exclude conditions better treated by other specialists.*   Some abnormal physical findings are indications of life-threatening or serious pathology which need to be referred appropriately.

*2.    To reassure the patient that the pain warrants no further investigation or surgery.*   This breaks the cycle of repeated investigation without findings to account for pain and unnecessary referral for further medical opinion.

*3.    To find physical signs associated with pain.*   Although visceral, neurological and orthopaedic components to pain have been investigated, signs of musculo-skeletal tenderness or sensory signs such as allodynia, hyperalgesia and hyperpathia are frequently missed until the pain clinic physician's examination. This may be because the significance of these signs has not been understood.

*4.    To define baseline signs and monitor changes.*   All physical signs should be documented at the outset to enable assessment of the effect of treatment or to allow monitoring of deterioration at subsequent physical examination.

*5.    As a specific search for inconsistencies between symptoms and findings on examination, or during examination in different positions.*   The presence of inconsistency does not imply 'exaggeration' or 'fraud'. It may simply indicate communication difficulties between different doctors or between doctor and patient. It is a reflection that in chronic pain, amplification of symptoms without obvious findings is to be expected. An example of this is the subjective sensation of swelling that can occur in many painful conditions but may have no objective signs.

## Back pain

### The back

1.   *Inspection*
- Scars.
- Muscle spasm.
- Structural or postural abnormalities.

## 2. Palpation
- Spinous processes.
- Area over facet joints.
- Paravertebral areas.

## 3. Range of movement
- Determination of restriction.
- Attention to provocation of pain: flexion of lumbar spine causing leg pain.
- Rotation or extension of spine provoking pain from posterior structures.

# Relevant neurological examination

Neurological examination distinguishes between back pain without root tension signs, back pain with simple root tension signs and back pain with neurological signs which need to be assessed by a surgeon. For thoracic back pain, wasting and sensory abnormalities of the trunk should be excluded. For all back pain, neurological assessment of the legs and perineum should be made as follows:

## 1. Nerve root tension signs
- Provocation of radicular pain by coughing or sneezing.
- Limited straight-leg raise. Each leg is examined separately. A positive finding on straight leg raise (SLR) is the reproduction of leg or buttock pain. The angle at which this occurs should be noted in degrees. SLR limited by the production of back pain does not necessarily imply nerve root tension. A SLR of less than 10° does not suggest nerve root tension.
- A positive sciatic stretch test is the exacerbation of radicular pain by dorsiflexion of the foot.
- Crossed leg pain is the provocation of pain in the symptomatic leg by straight raising of the other leg. It is highly suggestive of a prolapsed intervertebral disc.
- The finding of apparent tension in one position e.g. lying that is not reproduced in the sitting position has been described as an 'inappropriate' sign. The significance of the word 'inappropriate' is in relation to the diagnosis of disc irritation. It is regrettable that this inconsistency has been misinterpreted as implying that the patient is 'misleading' the clinician.

## 2. Muscle power is assessed by obvious wasting and grading of the following movements:
- Hip flexion dependent on L1 and L2 roots.
- Knee flexion dependent on L5, S1 and S2 roots.
- Knee extension dependent on L3 and L4 roots.
- Ankle plantar flexion dependent on S1 root.
- Ankle dorsiflexion dependent on L4 and L5 roots.
- Extension of the big toe dependent on L5 and S1 roots.

**3. *Sensation*** to cotton wool and/or pin prick should be determined according to whether deficiency is in a dermatomal, peripheral nerve or other distribution, such as glove and stocking or whole limb. There may be signs of hyperexcitability such as allodynia, hyperalgesia or hyperpathia.

**4. *Reflexes.*** Patellar and ankle reflexes imply intact L3/L4 and S1/S2 nerve roots respectively. Up-going plantars and hyper-reflexia need referral for the investigation of an upper motor neurone problem and lead the examiner to search for a motor, sensory and reflex level.

**5. *Nerve root signs.*** Compression of the S1 nerve root by the L5/S1 disc causes weakness of plantar flexion, reduced sensation in the S1 distribution and an absent or diminished ankle jerk. (Symmetrical loss of the ankle jerks is, however, common in the elderly without pathology.) Compression of the L5 nerve root by an L4/L5 disc causes weakness of the extensor hallucis longus, reduced sensation in the L5 distribution but may not result in changes in the reflexes. The findings of paraesthesia of legs and perineum, a lax anal sphincter, weakness of ankle movements with absent ankle reflexes in a patient with back pain requires urgent (same day) exclusion of an acute central disc prolapse, a surgical emergency.

# Neck pain

## The neck

### 1. Inspection
- Deformities.
- Scars.
- Muscle atrophy.
- Abnormal vertebral contour.

### 2. Palpation
- Tenderness.
- Muscle spasm.

### 3. Range of movement in all parameters
- Determination of restriction.
- Attention to provocation of pain.

## Relevant neurological examination

**1. *Muscle power*** is assessed by obvious wasting and grading of the following movements:

- Arm abduction dependent on C5 root.
- Elbow flexion dependent on C5 and C6 roots.
- Elbow extension dependent on C7 root.
- Wrist extension dependent on C6 root.
- Wrist flexion dependent on C7 root.
- Finger extension dependent on C7 root.
- Finger flexion and adduction dependent on C8 root.
- Finger abduction dependent on C8 and T1 roots.

**2. Sensation** is tested in the same way as in the legs during the neurological examination of the back. A common misdiagnosis of a sensory level is when it occurs in the arms – remember that C4 dermatome anteriorly can extend down the chest wall. High sensory level (foramen magnum) can also easily be missed – it occurs along the coronal suture!

**3. Reflexes**
- Normal biceps reflex implies intact C5 root.
- Normal brachioradialis reflex implies intact C6 root.
- Normal triceps reflex implies intact C7 root.

In cervical myelopathy reflexes may be brisk.

# Limb pain

## The limb

**1. Inspection**
- Deformity.
- Wasting.
- Discolouration.
- Oedema or trophic changes, such as loss of hair or shiny skin.

**2. Palpation**
- Tenderness.
- Muscle spasm.
- Temperature change can be noted by comparison with the opposite limb.

**3. Range of movement.** Passive and active movement (with quantification of its limitation) estimates function, particularly of a joint.

# Head and face pain

Physical examination within the pain clinic is to reinforce that the referral of a face pain or headache is appropriate and does not require other specialist input.

## Head and face

**1. Inspection**
- Face.
- Head.
- Inside of mouth.
- External auditory meatus.

**2. Palpation**
- Surface of head.
- Temporal arteries.
- Temporomandibular joints for tenderness and clicking on closure, areas of reported tenderness, trigger points or neuromata.
- Facial sinuses.

### Relevant neurological examination

- Neuralgias for nerve entrapment causing provocation of pain.
- Trigeminal sensory testing for deficiency and hyperexcitability.
- The presence of 'trigger' points.
- Cranial nerves (corneal reflex, visual fields and acuity, ocular movements), hearing, motor power.

### Occlusal analysis

- Interincisal distance should be three finger breadths and closure should be smooth.
- There should be no side-to-side deviation or midline shift as maximum closure is approached.

## Abdominal, pelvic and perineal pain

Visceral components of pain presenting to the pain clinic are usually seen by specialists in surgical and medical disciplines prior to referral. Superficial tenderness or sensory abnormality may however not have been noted. It is rarely appropriate to perform a rectal or vaginal examination. If appropriate this should be a chaperoned procedure.

## Related topics of interest

Assessment of chronic pain – history (p. 17); Back pain – medical management (p. 29).

# ASSESSMENT OF CHRONIC PAIN – PSYCHOSOCIAL

*Andrew Severn, Barrie Tait*

Chronic pain is a multifaceted experience and any assessment of it must consider the impact of the pain on the sufferer. To consider it as no more than an injury which has run a longer than usual course is to miss the diagnosis of the disease called chronic pain, or 'the chronic pain syndrome'. Many conditions may present acutely as minor injuries but symptoms do not resolve spontaneously for a variety of reasons. The pain experience can be described as having five dimensions:

- The sensation of pain.
- The patient's suffering and distress: the affective dimension.
- The patient's expectations and beliefs: the cognitive dimension.
- The patient's complaints or non-verbal communication: the behavioural dimension.
- The impact on the patient of the social environment.

Information about these is important in the assessment of the chronic pain sufferer. It is recommended that the contribution of psychosocial factors is considered at an early stage in non-specific low back pain. Psychosocial factors can be assessed systematically by looking specifically for certain attitudes, beliefs, behaviours and motivational factors. In the case of non-specific low back pain the clinician should be wary of the patient who takes the attitude that exercise will be impossible unless the pain is abolished, who relies on appliances, takes extensive rest, or whose expectation is that the professional will be able to cure the problem. These symptoms have been described as 'yellow flags': diagnostic screening aids to the presence of psychosocial dysfunction.

Psychosocial assessment can be left to professional psychology personnel in those clinics which have the luxury of these staff. Their absence from other clinics, however, does not mean that the task can be ignored. A variety of psychological screening tests are available: though designed for specialist psychological assessment by trained professionals, some of them are easily administered by the non-specialist. Most take the form of multiple-choice-type questions which can be completed by the patient in the clinic. Their value in the clinic that does not have psychological support is three-fold: they may help to identify the patient whose psychological scores are well outside the norm for the population and may thus be unsuitable for the limited expertise available in the clinic; they allow progress to be charted; and they allow colleagues to share information using a common language. On the other hand, there is evidence that the tests are not diagnostic on their own, and their use in quantifying the response to psychological treatments is disappointing.

In considering the psychosocial aspect, it is important for the clinician to distinguish between the multidimensional model and the concept of malingering. Illness behaviour is not a state of malingering nor even of conscious expression of disability. It is not a sign of abnormal psychological function, even though some of its more idiosyncratic manifestations may cause wonder and, occasionally, amusement. Illness behaviour is a normal part of the experience of chronic pain. Its manifestation is subject to the principles governing human behaviour: attention to a behaviour, or rewarding it (by sympathy or taking on chores), encourages a repetition of the behaviour.

## The subjective experience of pain

The nociceptive system for pain has, at the interface between the individual and the environment, nerve endings of simple structure whose physiological activity varies according to the local environment. The type of word used tells us something about the subjective experience of pain and its effect on the individual. The McGill scoring system offers a choice of words to describe the pain. Some of them (like 'aching' or 'burning') are straightforward symptoms suggesting nociceptive or neuropathic pain. Others imply a degree of central nervous system integration of inputs.

## Attitudes and beliefs

The traditional medical model explains the purpose of pain in that pain has a protective function, promoting rest of the injured part, and warning of environmental hazards. This is a belief that persists when someone suffers chronic pain after an injury. This belief is an important determinant of persistent disability. It is influenced by the way in which the injury is managed by the attending professionals. For example, someone to whom the word 'arthritis' is synonymous with a wheelchair-bound parent will be reluctant to exercise the spine that has been described to have 'arthritic changes'. Similarly, the inevitable and appropriate caution with which an ambulance paramedic and a hospital doctor treat a road accident victim with neck pain or the patient with angina may lead to a state of hypervigilance in which very minor symptoms assume great significance, long after the nociceptive causes for the pain have resolved. This is known as 'symptom expectation'. The belief that there is an ongoing nociceptive cause and a continuing disease is an important determinant of chronicity. This belief can be perpetuated by the professional adopting a purely biomedical view of the symptoms, such as continuing to look for a cause of the pain. Requests for investigations of increasing sophistication to find a cause for the pain are common, and compliance with these requests may reinforce the patient's view that there is a serious problem. Repeated radiological examination may occasionally be useful in demonstrating to the patient that there has been no progressive damage, but the clinician must make sure that the patient understands the purpose of the examination. In particular, it is worth noting that if a patient expects that a test will show an abnormality, a normal result may worsen the patient's distress.

## Suffering and distress

Depressive thoughts and loss of self esteem, even suicidal thoughts, are to be expected in a chronically painful condition. The premorbid state is relevant. In view of the common neurotransmitters involved in regulating mood and pain experience, there is good reason to view chronic pain and depression as diseases with features in common. There are several self-rating questionnaires which were developed for use in screening for depression but which have been successfully adapted for the chronic pain population. The hospital anxiety and depression index (HAD) and the modified Zung index are examples. 'Catastrophizing' is a technical term for 'fearing the worst' and refers to such emotions associated with thoughts such as 'I can't go on' or 'this pain is never going to get better'. It can, as part of a detailed psychological evaluation, be assessed in a quantitative way. 'Locus of control' is the technical term for the patient's view of the responsibility for pain management. The patient who looks to the professional for a cure is 'externally controlled', the one who is prepared to consider responsibility for self-management is 'internally controlled'.

## Illness behaviour

Illness behaviour is the way in which a sufferer communicates the experience of pain. In its simplest, most easily observed form, this can take the form of grimacing or complaint on examination. The display of such behaviour is not governed entirely by the activity of nociceptors, but is influenced by cultural and social factors. Thus the frequency of reports of chronic neck pain after vehicle trauma may not correlate with the frequency of crashes in a particular country, but may be influenced by factors such as the availability of affordable healthcare, the number of professionals available to treat the condition and the ease of access to the litigation process. Even simple clinical tools have the potential for producing illness behaviour, by drawing the sufferer's attention to the persistence of the condition. For example, keeping a diary of daily pain symptoms may lead to an inappropriate focusing on the persistence of these symptoms, a phenomenon known as 'symptom amplification'. It is worth seeing a number of presentations of chronic pain as 'illness behaviour'. Some patients wear cervical or lumbar supports in a way that makes their presence very visible. Transcutaneous nerve stimulators can easily be concealed in pockets, but some patients wear them in a way in which they can easily be seen. Even drugs have the potential for allowing illness behaviour to be demonstrated: the transdermal preparations of fentanyl or glyceryl trinitrate can be worn under clothing, but may be worn prominently on exposed skin. A bottle of analgesic tablets may be carried prominently in a jacket pocket. The observation of illness behaviour is sometimes taken as 'evidence' that the patient is consciously exaggerating the symptoms for personal gain. This may not be the case. A number of factors govern the presence of illness behaviour. In general terms illness behaviour will persist (be reinforced) as long as attention to the behaviour is made, and may disappear (be extinguished) if attention is not forthcoming. The professional may be unable to influence the way in which behaviour will be reinforced or extinguished in the patient's day-to-day life. Thus a patient who is excused normal domestic responsibilities because of chronic pain reporting may continue to wear a cervical collar despite professional advice not to do so.

## The social environment

Management of the chronic pain patient involves rehabilitating the patient back into a meaningful role in society. This may require a careful assessment of the work and social environment, so that activity, when it is resumed, is undertaken at a level compatible with ability. The financial factor is significant amongst social influences. The patient who stands to lose all financial benefits if he manages to overcome the powerful demotivating influences of cognitive, affective and behavioural complications of chronic pain may fall at the last hurdle unless this issue is addressed.

## Further reading

Ferrari R, Russell AS. Epidemiology of whiplash: an international dilemma. *Annals of the Rheumatic Diseases*, 1999; **58**: 1–5.

Kendal NAS, Linton SJ, Main CJ. *Guide to assessing psychosocial yellow flags in acute low back pain: risk factors for long-term disability and work loss.* Wellington, NZ: 1997. Accident Rehabilitation and Compensation Insurance Corporation of New Zealand and the National Health Committee, Ministry of Health, 1997; 1–22.

## Related topics of interest

Back pain – medical management (p. 29); Depression and pain (p. 73); Therapy – psychological (p. 195).

# BACK PAIN – MEDICAL MANAGEMENT

*Barrie Tait, Andrew Severn*

Low back pain currently accounts for more than half of all musculoskeletal disability; whilst work loss due to back pain in the UK is approximately 52 million days per year. Disability due to low back pain has reached epidemic proportions although there is no evidence for an increase in pathology. The cost of treating back pain is 1% of the total UK NHS budget. Assessment of the back pain sufferer establishes:

- Whether there is life-threatening disease.
- Whether there is nerve root involvement.
- Whether there is systemic disease.

It is intended that this assessment be carried out in the acute stage of initial presentation and at regular intervals thereafter. In many cases the diagnosis of non-specific low back pain can be made with confidence. Once this diagnosis has been achieved, further investigation is not required, unless there is a significant change in the pain.

## Serious or systemic disease

The following factors should alert to the possibility of serious or systemic disease. Features are referred to as 'red flags'. The reporting of such a symptom is a 'red flag' for the presence of a serious condition that needs investigation rather than symptomatic treatment or rehabilitation.

### 1. Symptoms of serious disease
- Bilateral or alternating symptoms.
- Constant or progressive pain.
- Night-time pain.
- Morning stiffness, relieved by exercise.
- Acute onset in the elderly.
- History of cancer.
- Fever or night sweats.
- Immunosuppression.
- Recent bacterial infection.
- Acute neurological symptoms, such as painful footdrop, perineal sensory impairment or sphincter disturbance.

### 2. Examination
- Tenderness on sacroiliac springing.
- Multiple nerve root signs suggesting compression over a number of lumbar segments from tumour or dissociative signs suggestive of intrinsic cord pathology.
- Symmetrical limitation of straight leg raising.
- Spinal rigidity, tenderness or deformity such as kyphus or step.
- Absent lower limb pulses or other features of lower limb ischaemia.
- Abdominal mass.

In the presence of red flags the following conditions should be considered as possible causes of back pain. The list is not exhaustive. This text will not discuss the investigation of the following:

- Aortic aneurysm.
- Retroperitoneal fibrosis.
- Tumour (primary or secondary).
- Gynaecological pathology.
- Ankylosing spondylitis.
- Metabolic bone disease.
- Infection.
- Osteoporosis.
- Paget's disease.
- Potts' disease.
- Myeloma.

Detailed discussion of investigation is beyond the scope of this book, but tests such as erythrocyte sedimentation rate (ESR), blood count, bone biochemistry, lumbar spine and sacroiliac joint X-ray or isotope bone scan can be easily organized in the pain clinic. Some clinics have access to magnetic resonance imaging and computed tomography that will provide more information.

## Back pain with nerve root involvement

With the proviso that the acute presentation of the cauda equina syndrome of perineal numbness, bilateral leg pain and sphincter disturbance described above is recognized as a 'red flag' necessitating immediate surgical referral, other nerve root symptoms and signs in the absence of 'red flags' can be treated symptomatically. Nerve root involvement may be treatable surgically. It is said that symptoms differ depending on whether nerve roots are irritated or compressed by disc or bony stenosis, being experienced as pain or numbness respectively. As a general rule, decompression is said to be more likely to be successful if it is carried out before the onset of numbness, which may be a late feature. Symptoms result from compression or irritation of the nerve root by either disc, bone or ligamentous hypertrophy. Symptoms and signs are of numbness and weakness in the appropriate dermatome and myotome, with loss of reflex at the corresponding root level and pain in the dermatome made worse by the manoeuvre of the sciatic or femoral stretch test.

Compression of the nerve root by a far lateral disc protrusion in the lateral foramen may cause diagnostic confusion with a high lumbar disc prolapse, with pain referred to the front of the thigh. However, the far lateral disc lesion may also be associated with muscle wasting due to direct compression of motor nerve roots that allows the differential diagnosis to be made on clinical grounds. Neurogenic claudication (pain on walking associated with spinal stenosis) may be confused with intermittent claudication of vascular origin, but distinguished from it by its slower recovery course and radicular distribution.

## Non-specific low back pain

The diagnosis of non-specific or 'idiopathic' low back pain is a diagnosis of exclusion. The optimal management is the subject of debate: some consider that it is not a medical problem and there is no medical solution. It must be considered in the wider context of functional and psychosocial factors, with an overall aim of reducing the disability as well as controlling symptoms.

If a diagnosis of non-specific low back pain is entertained further observations may be valuable in defining an anatomical origin. However, for reasons explained above, the search for relevant pathology may be fruitless. Although modern imaging techniques may provide a non-invasive and safe way of investigating back pain, the sensitivity of these techniques is such that the distressed patient may focus on minor abnormalities in a way that does not help management. In the case of, for example, minor alterations of the intervertebral disc, magnetic resonance imaging is said to demonstrate these in up to 30% of patients without symptoms. Certainly, attempts at symptomatic treatment and rehabilitation should not await the completion of such investigation. However easily available modern techniques for imaging are, it is imperative that the clinician does not forget that the decision to investigate carries with it the risk of undermining the patient's confidence in the clinical diagnosis. It may reinforce a belief that there is something seriously wrong. Prior discussion with a radiologist may avoid the danger of making too much of the presence of minor and inconsequential scan findings.

The site of the pain may be defined in terms of symptoms in two different ways: one way seeks to identify the anatomical location responsible according to symptoms, the other describes the spine as a series of segments. Both models have their uses in diagnosis and treatment.

## Specific anatomical syndromes

The suggestion that radiological changes in the lumbar zygoapophyseal (facet) joints indicate a cause for the pain was first entertained in 1911, but there is no correlation between the X-ray appearance and the degree of pain. The idea of a specific 'facet syndrome' as a clinical diagnosis is by no means universally accepted. Where it is used, however, it relates to a symptom complex that describes pain from the posterior structures of the vertebral column, and to be compared with other diagnoses.

1. *Facet syndrome*
- Continuous pain.
- Worsened by rotation and extension.
- Radiation into the leg, or the gluteal area, in a non-dermatomal distribution.
- Tenderness over the joints and paravertebral muscle spasm.

2. *Ligamentous pain*
- Pain worsened by flexion and extension.
- Tenderness is worse when the back muscles are relaxed.

### 3. Pain from vertebral body

- Back pain radiating to buttock and leg.
- Straight leg raising worsens the back pain but not the leg pain.

## Lumbar segmental dysfunction

This concept, an alternative one from that mentioned above considers that the spine is a series of bony segments connected by motion segments. Each *motion segment* therefore consists of part of the body of adjacent vertebrae, the intervertebral disc, the paired zygoapophyseal joints and the associated ligaments, capsules and muscles and fascia. All these structures have nociceptors, except for the nucleus pulposus and the inner two thirds of the annulus fibrosus, and therefore have the potential to be a site of origin of pain. The concept is a useful alternative to a fruitless search for non-existent pathology in the anatomical structures.

Lumbar segmental dysfunction is defined as lumbar pain, ostensibly due to excessive strains imposed on the restraining elements of a single spinal motion segment. The clinical features of lumbar segmental dysfunction are lumbar spinal pain, with or without referred pain that can be aggravated by selectively stressing a particular spinal motion segment. There is tenderness detectable locally and also at a distance in the areas of referred pain. Diagnostic confusion may be caused if it is not realized that autonomic changes may also occur.

*Diagnostic criteria.* All the following criteria should be satisfied:

- The affected motion segment must be specified.
- Pain is aggravated by clinical tests that selectively stress the affected motion segment.
- Stressing adjacent motion segments does not reproduce the patient's pain.

The diagnosis of segmental dysfunction is one step in establishing a possible site of origin of spinal pain. Because the innervation of a particular motion segment may be from more than one nerve, and because primary nociceptive fibres project widely onto spinal cord neurons, identification of a single lumbar segmental dysfunction may be difficult.

In practice the two concepts can be combined. For example, differential blocks of the medial branch of the dorsal spine, or the sinuvertebral nerve may further refine the diagnosis to the painful structure to posterior or anterior elements respectively. Further investigations might result in the patient's condition being ascribed a more definitive diagnosis, such as discogenic pain, or zygoapophyseal (facet) joint pain. The relevant investigations are injections of contrast medium into the intervertebral disc or the intra-articular space of the facet joint with the purpose of provoking discomfort from sites responsible for symptoms.

A precise structural diagnosis is not always possible, but the diagnosis of lumbar segmental dysfunction does allow physical and injection treatments to be more specifically directed.

## Management of acute and chronic back pain

The optimum management of 'idiopathic' back pain thus remains a controversial issue. It is clear that there is no one 'correct' way of treating the symptoms. In practice many patients will be prescribed paracetamol/codeine preparations, anti-inflammatory drugs, and some will claim that opioids alone provide sufficient relief for normal activity to be undertaken. The key to successful management is one of looking at the symptoms within a broader context of reduction of disability and tackling beliefs about the nature and significance of the spinal pain. This requires a multidisciplinary approach with a similar aim. As far as published evidence from systematic reviews is concerned, there is extensive literature whose findings are here summarized, with injection therapy and surgery being discussed in other chapters.

- *Acupuncture* has not been shown to be superior to 'sham acupuncture', where needles are placed randomly, for the treatment of low back pain.
- *Antidepressants.* Their value in back pain remains unproven.
- *Anti-inflammatory drugs.* The value of NSAIDs for the short-term treatment of acute low back pain has been demonstrated.
- *Back schools.* The effectiveness of this particular approach, which consists of an education and skills programme with an exercise regime has been demonstrated. The benefits are experienced over 3–6 months only, and are best achieved in the context of an intensive programme in a specialist centre. The value of an occupational setting for the school is believed to be of value.
- *Bed rest* delays recovery and return to work in acute back ache. Patients who stay in bed report no less pain at later follow up compared with those who stay active. It is no better to stay in bed for seven days than it is for two to three days.
- *Behavioural therapy.* The value of behavioural therapy in reducing the disability and improving the understanding of back pain has been shown. Some reports of reduction in pain intensity have also been shown.
- *Group education* as a single treatment provided short-term reduction in pain intensity in one of four studies of patients with chronic back ache, and in one of two studies of patients with acute back ache, in which it reduced sick leave duration.
- *Exercise therapy.* The value of specific exercise therapy, as opposed to conventional physiotherapy treatments or conservative management for acute back pain has not been demonstrated. However, it may be helpful in the chronic setting, as part of a programme to return to normal activity and work.
- *Physical therapy.* Manual therapy for acute back ache may be effective in patients with radiating pain and recurrent pain. The evidence in favour of massage, used in a number of trials as a control treatment, is uncertain.

# Further reading

Back Pain. *Report of a CSAG Committee on Back Pain* (Chaired by M. Rosen). London: HMSO, 1994.
Cohen JE *et al.* Group education interventions for people with low back pain: an overview of the literature. *Spine*, 1994; **19:** 1214–22.

## Systematic reviews

Evans G, Richards S. *Low back pain: an evaluation of therapeutic interventions.* University of Bristol, Health Care Evaluation Unit; p. 176.

Koes BW, Vantulder MW, Vanderwindt DAWM, Bouter LM. The efficacy of back schools: a review of randomised clinical trials. *Journal of Clinical Epidemiology,* 1994; **47**: 851–2.

Turner JA, Denny MC. Do antidepressant medications relieve chronic low back pain? *Journal of Family Practice,* 1993; **37**: 545–53.

## Related topics of interest

Assessment of chronic pain – psychosocial (p. 25); Back pain – injections (p. 35); Back pain – surgery (p. 40); Musculoskeletal pain syndromes (p. 95); Therapy – anti-inflammatory drugs (p. 162); Therapy – physical (p. 193); Therapy – psychological (p. 195).

# BACK PAIN – INJECTIONS

*Andrew Severn, Barrie Tait*

There are several targets for intervention techniques in the treatment of back pain. There are many nerve pathways implicated in the experience of back pain, and as many enthusiasts for one particular technique as there are uncontrolled reports of efficacy. The treatment of back pain has, however, to be seen in the light of other factors that influence its occurrence and prognosis. The disability caused by back pain is out of proportion to pathology. Patients with psychological distress or illness behaviour may have unrealistic expectations of treatment. Nerve blocks should be seen as part of a process of education and rehabilitation, allowing an opportunity for mobilization and return to normal activity.

## Anatomy

Posterior structures of the motion segment are innervated by the dorsal primary ramus of the spinal nerve. The structures are:

- Facet joints.
- Posterior part of the dura.
- Ligaments.
- Back muscles.

Anterior structures are innervated by a nerve plexus (the sinuvertebral nerve) which enters the spinal nerve in the sympathetic communicating ramus and projects to several levels of the spinal cord. The structures are:

- Vertebral bodies.
- Longitudinal ligaments.
- Discs.
- Anterior part of the dura.
- Paravertebral muscles.

## Nerve blocks as a diagnostic tool

Differential blocks of the medial branch of the dorsal spine, or the sinuvertebral nerve may refine a diagnosis of lumbar segmental dysfunction to the painful structure to posterior or anterior elements. Further investigations might result in the patient's condition being ascribed a more definitive diagnosis, such as discogenic pain, or zygoapophyseal (facet) joint pain. The relevant investigations are injections of contrast medium into the intervertebral disc or the intra-articular space of the facet joint with the purpose of provoking discomfort from sites responsible for symptoms. However, as far as selective nerve block is concerned, in view of the diffuse projections of the sinuvertebral nerve, only the nerve supply to the facet joints (and it has to be remembered that they receive additional innervation from the dorsal primary ramus of the adjacent nerve root immediately above and below) can be considered specific in terms of localizing the anatomical source of the pain.

## Nerve blocks as targets for nerve lesions and therapeutic injections

Only the medial branch of the dorsal primary ramus can be described as providing a specific sensory supply to one particular part of the spine, in this case the facet joint. The anterior structures do not lend themselves to specific nerve block so easily. However, nociceptive stimuli from the intervertebral discs can be reduced by radiofrequency nerve lesioning technique in which the heat transfer through the disc causes a lesion in the adjacent sinuvertebral nerve. In all the considerations the proximity of the mixed spinal nerve must be remembered, and appropriate stimulation test undertaken to ensure that it is not subjected to a nerve block or a lesion.

Although a score or so of randomized controlled trials now exist conerning the efficacy of spinal injections for back pain, one systematic review has commented on the poor quality of the design of many trials of injections for back pain. The difficulty in designing controlled studies lies partly with the multitude of factors that complicate the presentation of back pain, and the many outcome measures that can be undertaken. Patients with relapsing symptoms may require a multidisciplinary approach to rehabilitation, and a cure of symptoms with repeated injections may not be achievable.

## Techniques

*1. **Steroid injections.*** Steroid injections around or into the facet joint are common pain clinic interventions. Preference for the injection target varies and there is no consensus about the optimal dose or timing of the procedure. Systematic review has identified three randomized trials which have attempted to answer whether facet joint steroid injections are useful. One of these took a group of patients who had previously responded to local anaesthetic block of the facet joints, and then compared a steroid injection procedure with placebo control to show a possible beneficial effect at 6 months. One compared two different injection techniques (into the facet joint capsule and around the facet joint capsule) with placebo, failing to show a difference between the two groups. The third compared two common interventions: block of the nerve to the facet joint with an intra-articular steroid joint injection and claimed a beneficial effect for both techniques, but did not include a placebo group. Any of these results can be used to justify the various approaches to facet joint injection with or without steroid and give little firm guidance as to the most effective technique. In respect of duration of pain relief it is difficult to refuse repeated injections for the patient who responds to injection with an improvement of mobility and reduction of pain symptoms that lasts a few weeks.

The rationale for the use of steroids in the epidural space is the presence of inflammation around nerve roots. Many reports and observational studies claiming benefit for epidural steroids pre-dated the systematic study with controlled trials. Two systematic reviews have been undertaken. One has found six randomized controlled trials supporting the use of epidural steroids for the short-term treatment of back pain with leg pain, and an equal number of trials failing to conclude the same. By pooling results from randomized controlled trials, a second review has calculated NNT of epidural steroids of 7 for 75% pain relief at 60 days and 13 for 50% at one year. There is controversy surrounding the use of epidural steroids, however, not least in view of some of the claims that have been made for them, and for intrathecal steroids. Historically epidural and intrathecal steroids have been used for a number of conditions, and recently suggested in the management of postherpetic neuralgia. In common with many drugs used by pain clinicians, depot steroids do not have a product licence for epidural use. Indeed, advice has been given in the past that epidural steroids, even correctly administered, should not be used because of neurotoxicity. (This advice was based on anecdotal Australian reports that were never substantiated.) One manufacturer actively discourages the practice of epidural injection by printing warnings on the ampoule. Of concern is the presence of benzylalcohol and/or polyethylene glycol, a non-ionic detergent in the pharmaceutical preparation. The risk of accidental administration into the subarachnoid space should be considered: methyl prednisolone can cause arachnoiditis if so injected. Every effort should be made to ensure that the drug is deposited outside the dura. As with facet joint injections, there is no consensus on the practice of repeated epidural injections for relapsing symptoms and it is difficult to deny any patient who derives relief measured in weeks, as indeed is the finding in some of the controlled trials. The possibility of a cumulative effect of repeated steroid administration is one factor that may influence practice.

Paravertebral and dorsal root ganglion injections are variants of the epidural steroid injection, targeting specific nerve roots. Under X-ray control, contrast medium can occasionally be seen entering the epidural space. The same considerations therefore apply as for the use of long-acting steroids.

**2.   *Radiofrequency nerve lesions.*** It is convenient to describe a hierarchy of procedures that can be carried out with radiofrequency lesioning. These progress from the most simple, least invasive to the more invasive. The technique chosen will be determined by the likely diagnosis supported by appropriate diagnostic local anaesthetic tests. The heirarchy has been described as (in increasing order of technical difficulty):

- Facet joint lesion (medial branch of primary dorsal ramus).
- Lumbar sympathetic chain lesion.
- Lumbar disc lesion.
- Lesion of the communicating ramus.
- Lesion of the dorsal root ganglion.

The value of radiofrequency lesioning of medial branch of the primary dorsal ramus of the segmental nerve has been demonstrated in a randomized controlled trial on patients who had previously responded to a block of the nerve with local anaesthetic. The nerve is blocked where it crosses the superior surface of the transverse process of the lumbar vertebra. X-ray imaging is required for localization. The needle must not travel anterior to the transverse process or the mixed spinal nerve will be blocked as it emerges from the spinal foramen. The absence of motor stimulation is an additional confirmatory test that must be performed before lesioning.

When performing a destructive lesion the needle position is checked first by stimulating the nerve and checking that the mixed spinal nerve is not being stimulated. The contribution of fibres from the joint above should be considered when the procedure is performed.

Lumbar sympathetic chain and communicating ramus lesions have been described for pain which involves the pathways of the sympathetic system and sinu-vertebral nerve. This is pain from the anterior structures of the spine, again assessed by history and the response to local anaesthetic block.

The same nerve pathways may be lesioned in lumbar disc lesions. In this technique, the radiofrequency probe is inserted into the disc. The thermal conductivity of the disc material and the lack of vascularity to the disc results in a gradient of temperature across the disc, with an effect on the nociceptors of the annulus fibrosus.

The dorsal root ganglion contains the cell bodies of primary afferent nociceptors and of larger, faster conducting fibres serving modalities of touch and vibration sense. The technique of dorsal root ganglion lesion carries with it the risk of causing damage to these latter neurons, resulting in anaesthesia of the skin. This risk is reduced by the use of a lower temperature for lesioning fibres, thereby causing a selective action on the unmyelinated small nociceptor neurons. A specific technique that allows this, lower temperature lesion, is pulsed radiofrequency current.

**3. *Imaging techniques for therapy.*** The use of a radiographic contrast medium in the epidural space can demonstrate scarring lesions around the nerves of the cauda equina. This technique enables the operator to observe the nerve root during injection of drugs into the epidural space, to target the drug to the radiological lesion and free the nerve from scar tissue by a hydrostatic pressure effect. The use of saline, local anaesthetic, steroids, hyaluronidase and hypertonic saline has been reported. A refinement of the technique involves the introduction of a fine catheter into the epidural space and its positioning adjacent to a scarred nerve root, with the aim of drug delivery near the suspected site of nerve injury. The space can also be inspected directly with the aid of a small fibre-optic instrument introduced via the sacral hiatus. This technique allows targeted injections and hydrostatic distension of scarred nerve roots under minimal sedation.

## Systematic reviews

Koes BW, Scholten RJPM, Mens JMA, Bouter LM. Efficacy of epidural steroid injections for low back pain and sciatica: a systematic review of randomized clinical trials. *Pain*, 1995; **63:** 279–88.

Nelemans PJ, Bie RA de, Vet HCW. Injection therapy for subacute and chronic benign low back pain. *Cochrane Library*, Issue 4, 2000.

Watts RW, Silagy CA. A meta-analysis on the efficacy of epidural corticosteroids in the treatment of sciatica. *Anaesthesia and Intensive Care*, 1994; **23:** 564–9.

## Further reading

Stolker RJ, Vervest ACM, Groen GJ. The management of chronic spinal pain by blockades: a review. *Pain*, 1994; **58:** 1–20.

## Related topics of interest

Back pain – medical management (p. 29); Therapy – nerve blocks: somatic and lesion techniques (p. 179).

# BACK PAIN – SURGERY

*Paul Eldridge*

This chapter is intended as a brief review of spinal surgery; it consists of an account of two categories of condition: those which comprise the majority of the practice of spinal surgery and a number of other conditions which though rare present with axial pain. Being rare the evidence for the management of such conditions is largely anecdotal, and based on basic surgical principles.

As it is an immense subject in its own right the problems of rheumatoid arthritis, ankylosing spondylitis and scoliosis are not mentioned here.

## Lumbar disc disease

The vast majority of spinal surgery is performed for lumbar disc prolapse. The incidence of lumbar disc degeneration is so high as to consider it a normal part of the ageing process. Often it will be asymptomatic, even when prolapse has occurred. In post-mortem studies of asymptomatic individuals the rate of prolapse is 15%. MRI scans cannot therefore be relied on to make a diagnosis of symptomatic anatomical abnormality, and much trouble ensues if the patient is made aware of normal degenerative changes without being made aware of their lack of clinical significance. Disc disease may present with either or both of low back pain or radicular symptoms. The former is due to the direct damage to the disc, whilst the latter to the effects of the disc protrusion itself. Low back pain is discussed elsewhere but suffice it to mention it may arise from sources other than the disc such as the muscles, ligaments, facet joints or the dural tube itself – this is not an exhaustive list.

### Disc prolapse

These may be considered to be contained or sequestered. The latter means that the nucleus of the disc has burst through the annulus. The earliest description of surgery for disc disease was by Dandy in 1921 (readers will remember he also first described microvascular decompression for trigeminal neuralgia) though the paper of Mixter and Barr in 1934 launched disc surgery.

### 'Typical'

The most common presentation of disc prolapse is radicular pain, i.e. sciatica. It may be preceded by a back strain or injury; and with an initial acute low back pain which settles to be replaced by sciatica. If the pain radiates below the knee in a dermatomal distribution then it is highly likely to be radicular in origin, though this is not an absolute rule. It is often associated with motor and sensory deficit relevant to the level of the prolapse; there should be root tension signs such as limitation of straight leg raise. 95% of disc prolapse occurs at L4/5 or L5/S1 and the presenting signs will give some indication of the level although not reliably enough to confirm the level for a surgical approach.

## Central

One of two variants of the presentation of lumbar disc prolapse, important because of its dire neurological consequences if missed, a central disc prolapse results in neurological deficit in the cauda equina, which may cause loss of function of bowel control, bladder control and sexual function. Saddle anaesthesia is typical, and sufficient nerves may be affected to result in lower motor neurone weakness of the lower limbs hence difficulty walking in addition to the effects of the pain. Pain is usual, and may include sciatic elements as well as the central cauda equina features. Disc decompression must be undertaken as an emergency. With this condition and with the more usual disc prolapse the contribution of lumbar spinal stenosis may be as significant as the disc prolapse itself.

## Far lateral

This syndrome is becoming increasingly recognized with the advent of cross-sectional imaging, in particular MR. The disc prolapse is outside the spinal canal – truly 'far lateral'. There may be a previous history of back injury, and complaint is of sharp back pain followed by pain in the hip and the anterior thigh. There may be associated weakness of the quadriceps. Its recognition is important; firstly so as not to miss structural pathology as a cause of the low pain and secondly as the surgical approach is different – unsurprisingly it is usually lateral!

## Investigations

In virtually all situations this is by MR imaging though occasionally myelography, usually with CT assistance is required. One obvious indication is when the patient is intolerant of MR due to claustrophobia; otherwise it may be used when clinical history and signs convince the clinician but the imaging does not! This reflects the fact that there are no good studies validating myelography – the previous standard – against MRI. The impact of non-invasive imaging is so as to render the role of examination of the patient more to confirm the clinical meaning of the findings on imaging than to attempt precise diagnosis of level or process.

## Treatment

It should not be forgotten that the natural history of sciatica due to disc prolapse is for it to resolve, although this may take some considerable time. In one study it has been claimed that there was no difference in symptoms of sciatica ten years after surgery comparing an operated with a non-operated group. One further interesting statistic is that the rate of operation for lumbar disc surgery is 100/100000 in the UK but this rises to 900/100000 in the US where there is abundant provision of the facilities for the investigation and surgical treatment of this condition. However, 90% of attacks of sciatica will settle conservatively; if a second attack occurs then the likelihood of remaining attack-free in the future falls to 50% and is further reduced with subsequent attacks. The risk of recurrent attacks also increases if the protrusion is not contained. Thus there is some evidence to confirm the clinical impression of neurosurgeons that large sequestered disc prolapses do cause recurrent severe episodes of sciatica, do well surgically, and that patients should therefore be advised with confidence that microdiscectomy is currently the best option.

The gold standard for treatment is microdiscectomy and is effective in over 90% in providing relief of sciatica. In perhaps 50% of cases back pain will be improved. The results are less good when recovery of neurological function is considered. This is important when the cauda equina is at risk, but the impact of a persistent foot drop should not be underestimated. The chance of recovery depends on the time for which function has been lost and this is why decompression for central disc is performed as an emergency. It is said that the chance of neurological recovery is better when pain is still present.

The operative philosophy is to minimize structural damage to the spine so a unilateral muscle strip is performed and a small fenestration made in the interlaminar space. The success rate is related to the degree of prolapse and those patients with 'negative explorations' do poorly. The use of the microscope has been associated with reduced hospital stay, and less denervation of paraspinal muscles when compared to open procedures, though an open procedure with full laminectomy may be necessary to provide safe access to large central disc protrusions. Occasionally the only way to obtain safe access to a central lumbar disc prolapse may be to go transdurally and remove a fragment by separating the nerves of the cauda equina. A popular patient misconception is that the whole disc is removed – in fact only the part comprising the protrusion is removed with perhaps some further amount from the disc space. Disc weights indicate that the average volume of disc removed is only 6–8% of the total. Surgery does not come without risk. There is a mortality rate (though low) due to thrombo-embolism, but there may also be infection including discitis. Epidural fibrosis may be one of the causes, not the only one for a chronic pain state – the failed back syndrome. Other treatments have been attempted for contained disc prolapse including chymopapain injection, percutaneous nucleotomy, and laser microdiscectomy. None of these have found wide acceptance; in the case of percutaneous nucleotomy a prospective randomized controlled trial showed it to be inferior to microdiscectomy. Chymopapain is dangerous if mistakenly injected into the sub-arachnoid space. There are no controlled randomized data regarding laser treatments as shown by its failure to gain acceptance.

## Neurogenic claudication and lumbar spinal stenosis

As the name suggests this presents as pain made worse on walking. Typically the pain is radicular, and takes about 10–15 min to resolve. These two features distinguish it from arterial claudication. Examination in the clinic is often normal again in contrast to arterial claudication. One feature of the history that is occasionally mentioned is that symptoms improve as the patient bends forward, for example to rest on a neighbour's garden gate after a fixed walking distance.

Investigation is by MRI, though if this fails then CT myelography may be used. The natural history is for the condition to be relatively stable so that conservative treatment after making the diagnosis is adequate. The conventional surgical treatment is by laminectomy and decompression though recently there is a trend to more conservative operations – multilevel fenestrations and undercutting facetectomy. This is because of the fear of destabilizing the back, though in practice this seldom happens.

In some circumstances medical treatment may be required. This is not as effective as the surgical treatment and is reserved for patients unfit for surgery, or those unwilling to accept surgery. The anticonvulsants may be tried – sodium valproate or carbemazepine or as an alternative calcitonin. Variably these attempts may produce success for a year or so.

## Low back pain

Critical analysis of surgery for low back pain is not encouraging. Since this is a surgical chapter no reference is made to the psychological aspects of the problem except to note that these are of great importance – and dealt with elsewhere in this volume.

When discectomy is performed purely for back pain the results are not good. There is much written regarding the role of spinal fusion with or without concomitant stabilization, and many major operations have been carried out for back pain on the basis that this is due to an 'unstable' back which can therefore be corrected by spinal stabilization. There is much energy invested in the design and production of different types of instrumentation, and in addition image-guided fluoroscopic techniques for safe placement of said instrumentation. However randomized trials, which are few in number, have not demonstrated any benefit from such operations and the popularity has therefore declined for such procedures in the UK though in North America the practice continues. Again, as with disc surgery the operation rate is much higher in the US than in UK at 80 compared to 15 per 100 000. If it is assumed that the spectrum of pathology is broadly similar then widely differing sets of indications for surgery must exist.

Currently a trial of intra-discal electrotherapy for back pain is being undertaken; this seems to amount to a disc denervation procedure so previous experience of procedures for pain relief would not lead to optimism as to the outcome of such a trial.

There continues to be interest in the use of spinal cord stimulation for low back pain. It is frequently observed that in cases stimulated for leg pain – usually failed back syndrome – the associated low back pain improves also. However despite enthusiasm this indication lacks proof of efficacy.

## Spondylolisthesis

This describes the situation where there is forward slip of one vertebra on another. In many instances it is asymptomatic but when it presents it is usually with back pain. The back pain is aggravated by activity and relieved by rest. The slip may also cause nerve root compression and therefore leg pain. Occasionally fusion is advised – principally in a younger age group (<35 years) but usually conservative treatment is the rule, contact sports being avoided in the young age group. Decompression of the nerve root is helpful for leg pain especially in patients over the age of 35 years in whom progression of slip is unlikely. This can be done by a 'microdisc' approach.

## Failed back surgery syndrome

An emotive expression describing the situation where there is persistence of symptoms following low back surgery. The incidence is about 5–10%. Of these perhaps as many as 15% may represent recurrent disc prolapse, and 50–60% be due to unrecognized lateral recess stenosis. Perhaps 20% are due to epidural fibrosis or arachnoiditis, and it is these cases that are of interest to the pain clinician. In parenthesis it is worth noting that these cases may respond well to spinal cord stimulation especially where leg pain is the predominant feature. Clearly the high incidence of structural and surgically remediable problems requires thorough investigation by imaging of failed back cases, and consideration for surgery. One difficult situation is where there is a combination of fibrosis and disc recurrence. Even with modern imaging it can be difficult to resolve this dilemma.

## Thoracic disc

This is a very rare syndrome with an incidence of only 1/1 000 000. Presenting features are back pain, radicular pain in an intercostal distribution and thoracic myelopathy. However pain is not the predominant feature and signs and symptoms of myelopathy are more common. Surgical excision is the treatment and this may involve a transthoracic approach.

## Tumours

### Intrinsic cord lesions

Intrinsic tumours of the spinal cord are rare; presentation is by neurological deficit in the main though a dull aching axial pain is often present. Because of the rarity of the condition diagnosis is made only after several months or even years. Occasionally (and see also *syringomyelia*) the neurological deficit may involve insensitivity to pain. Some tumours may be associated with central cord cysts, and this situation is sometimes classified as a type of syringomyelia. Treatment of the tumours is by biopsy and if possible surgical resection; occasionally this resection may be followed by central spinal cord neuropathic pain. Depending on the histology radiotherapy may be offered.

### Extrinsic cord compression

In the region of the conus, lesions such as ependymoma or neurofibroma cause a continuous and progressive pain. Clinically the pain is out of proportion to the signs and demeanour of the patient. Patients may get the label of exhibiting abnormal illness behaviour because of the distress and the lack of corresponding clinical signs. Such conditions can only be diagnosed by imaging, but it is important that the patient is aware of the indication for this. It is important to have an understanding that if investigation fails to demonstrate pathology subsequent treatment should be aimed at the distress and behaviour.

Meningioma, typically found in middle-aged women in the mid-thoracic zone, rarely presents with pain, typical findings being progressive paraparesis.

### Tumours of the spinal column

Apart from extremely rare primary bone tumours most lesions are metastatic. Pain may be of two types, with different treatment consequences. Instability pain arises when bone destruction by the metastasis renders the spine mechanically unstable. Pain is worse on movement, and refractory to analgesics whatever their potency. In these circumstances spinal fixation may be indicated. Secondly the pain may be continuous and represent the direct effect of the tumour; in this situation it is usually steroid responsive in the short-term and radiotherapy is effective. In recent years this presentation of metastatic tumour has become much rarer perhaps due to earlier detection by imaging and treatment by radiotherapy.

### Syrinx

A cavity in the spinal cord which may be as a result of tumour, trauma or Arnold–Chiari malformation. One of a number of conditions that may cause central spinal cord pain – a situation analogous to central post-stroke pain. Although treatment of the syrinx (shunting or third ventriculostomy for hydrocephalus, hind brain decompression or direct shunting of the syrinx itself) is necessary to prevent disease progression, pain is rarely relieved. Treatment must then be medical, but this is a difficult pain condition to manage.

## Infections

A number of infections may present with spinal pain. All are rare in the UK. Acute pyogenic infection, usually causing epidural abcess, causes severe local spinal pain, and the severity of the pain may suggest this diagnosis. Pain from tuberculosis is less acute and is more often related to instability due to the destructive nature of the condition.

Herpes zoster may present with spinal and dermatomal pain. Although the diagnosis is easy to make once vesicles have appeared in a segmental distribution it may be missed before this feature has appeared.

## Haematoma

Spinal sub-arachnoid haemorrhage occurs but is very rare. It can be due to spinal arteriovenous malformation (AVM) and this may have associated aneurysms. It presents with ictus, and in addition to spinal pain there may be radicular pain and meningism. Interestingly similar symptoms are sometimes seen following cranial aneurysmal subarachnoid haemorrhage, but not as the principal feature of the condition.

## Further reading

Porter RW, Miller CG. Neurogenic claudication and root claudication treated with calcitonin: a double blind controlled trial. *Spine*, 1988; **13**: 1061–4.

## Systematic reviews

Gibson JNA, Wadell G, Grant JC. *Surgery for degenerative lumbar spondylosis (Cochrane Review)*, The Cochrane Library, Issue 4, 2000, Oxford: Update Software.

Gibson JNA, Wadell G, Grant JC. *Surgery for lumbar disc prolapse (Cochrane Review)*, The Cochrane Library, Issue 4, 2000 Oxford: Update Software.

## Related topic of interest

Back pain – medical management (p. 29).

# BURNS

*Kate Grady, Andrew Severn*

The distinction of the acute pain state from the chronic pain state is one which is discussed in other chapters in this book. Chronic pain is well considered a disease, with its own natural history and presentation, its own treatments and techniques, whereas acute pain is a simpler model and is more easily understood by a person with a conventional biomedical training. There are, however, a few areas in clinical practice where the biology and the psychology of both acute and chronic pain states must be considered simultaneously and burn injury is one such area. Observation of the way in which casualties of the Anzio invasion force of 1944 viewed their serious wounds influenced the development of the model for pain pathways that we call the 'gate control' model. On a battlefield the prospect of a safe transfer, with honour, from a place of danger to a place of safety has been said to contribute to a sense of wellbeing, even analgesia. By contrast, in civilian practice, burn casualties might be considered the most extreme example of the way in which the circumstances contribute to adverse psychological outcomes, as the gate control mechanism may not work. Burn injuries are not only physically very painful, they are associated with devastating endocrine and metabolic changes, physical changes are often permanent, and psychological consequences of, for example, facial disfigurement, or the circumstances of the incident have to be considered from the very early stages.

It is recognized too that the transition from acute to chronic pain is a process of chemical and molecular change that we call neuroplasticity. The physiological processes and chemicals involved in burn injury themselves alter the behaviour of the neurones of the dorsal horn of the spinal cord, resulting in changes in pain sensitivity. Burns have the potential for releasing most of the inflammatory mediators and mediators producing sensitization and excitation of nociceptors and intense nociceptive input that is required to produce central sensitization, a process that has been described in the laboratory setting as 'windup'. The process of dressing changes and surgery results in further trauma, and each episode of nociceptive insult to the spinal cord has the potential for provoking further changes in the behaviour of the dorsal horn neurone. The constant threat, anticipation and experience of pain, together with the modelling from examples from history, may further exacerbate the psychological distress, as well as decreasing the threshold for pain. Animal evidence on postburn hyperalgesia, central hyperexcitability and changes in opioid sensitivity suggests that burns patients may need to be protected from developing a 'memory' of pain in neural networks.

## Pain during the immediate post-burn period and during intensive management

Pain is due to the acute and ongoing pain from the burn itself and due to measures undertaken to care for the burn and prevent its complications. Full thickness burns, even though the burnt area may be anaesthetic due to destruction of peripheral nociceptors must be considered a source of pain, as, of course, must the surrounding area where there may be less tissue damage, but intense stimulation of nociceptors. Pain in the acute period can be considered as two separate entities: a constant background pain and pain arising out of interventions such as dressings. Although strong opioid drugs are the mainstay of treatment, pain of intervention can be excruciating and inadequately controlled pharmacologically. It is accepted that there is a need for better analgesia for burn dressing changes. In this respect it is to be noted that paracetamol, nonsteroidal anti-inflammatory drugs (NSAIDs) or cycloxygenase II inhibitors (COXIBs), ketamine and other NMDA anatagonists, nitrous oxide, antidepressants and anticonvulsants are often used. It is also of note that one of the largest studies of the effects of opioid safety in respect of addiction potential was undertaken on military mass burn casualties, where it was concluded that opioids used for this purpose did not lead to addiction.

Topical lignocaine 2% has been applied to skin donor sites and has been shown to reduce opioid requirements. It has also been reported as effective in partial thickness burns, while intravenous lignocaine by infusion has also been reported of value. Benzodiazepines are often used as adjuncts. Lorazepam 1 mg has been reported to bring about a significant reduction in a high level of baseline pain.

Non-pharmacological interventions play an important part in the control of pain. Various cognitive, behavioural, relaxation, hypnotherapeutic and neuropsychological adjuncts have been used.

### Pain persisting into the rehabilitation period

There are many mechanisms that could be reasonably expected to perpetuate the sensitized status of the dorsal horn. These include the presence of continuing low-grade noxious stimulation, the presence of nerve damage, the disordered regeneration of nerve endings into scar tissue, and the presence of a degree of central nervous system sensitization at cortical level.

The return of abnormal skin sensation is common after burn injuries and many patients complain of painful sensations and paraesthesiae in their wounds. Tactile, thermal and pain thresholds have been found to be higher in areas of burns than in non-burned patients. Deep burns injuries are more affected than superficial burns. Sensory losses were found in burned and non-burned areas suggesting that the burned areas influence sensory perception in adjacent undamaged areas.

Patients are in the long term affected by intense itching. It is distressing and can compromise healing of newly formed fragile skin. It can occur at all stages of burn injury from 5 days to 2 years post burn, and occurs in wounds of any thickness and in donor sites. Antihistamines are used although they are not very effective. Non-pharmacological methods comprise control of ambient temperature, cool compresses, bathing, use of emollients, application of pressure, massage and the use of TENS.

Painful musculoskeletal problems may arise from deformities secondary to amputations, altered biomechanics or contractures.

## Related topics of interest

# CANCER – INTRATHECAL AND EPIDURAL INFUSIONS

*Kate Grady*

Intrathecal and epidural infusions (collectively known as spinal infusions in the practice of palliative care) are used not only in cancer pain but also in acute pain and selected benign chronic pains. In chronic benign pain appropriate patient selection is very important because there is the potential for serious side-effects and the long-term effects are not known. The importance of long-term commitment of both patient and physician should not be underestimated.

The principle of these routes of delivery is that small doses of analgesic drug are deposited in relatively high local concentrations, near to a spinal site of analgesic action. The need for systemic administration of drug is eliminated or reduced allowing sparing of systemic doses and consequent reduction in side-effects. The delivery of two synergistically acting drugs allows further sparing of dosage. Worldwide it is estimated that 3–5% of cancer patients could benefit from this mode of administration although as the techniques become more widely practiced, the relative indication for these routes as opposed to others with their side-effects, may become stronger.

Indications for these infusions are:

- Uncontrolled nociceptive pain, despite adequate trials of drugs by other routes.
- Uncontrolled neuropathic pain, despite adequate trials of drugs by other routes.
- Intolerable side-effects such as drowsiness or hallucinations from the use of drugs by other routes making their continued use unacceptable.
- To allow a short period of respite from high-dose opioids in cases of apparent opioid resistance.

Contraindications are:

- Lack of patient consent.
- Coagulopathy (consider in the presence of liver disease).
- Local sepsis or septicaemia.
- Very limited life expectancy.

The relative merits of each route have to be considered in deciding between intrathecal or epidural infusions.

## Advantages of epidural infusions

- Placement of an epidural line is technically easier.
- There is no leak of cerebrospinal fluid.
- Infection rates are lower.

## Advantages of intrathecal infusions

- A smaller volume and dose of injectate is required so there is less systemic uptake of drug.
- Segmental analgesia is not a problem.

- Smaller volumes make it possible to use implanted reservoir systems as part of the technique.
- If infection is suspected, cerebrospinal fluid (CSF) can be sampled for microbiological investigation.

## Drugs

Although the use of drugs for an unlicensed purpose is common practice in treatment of chronic and malignant pain it should not be undertaken lightly. With the exception of bupivacaine no drugs are licensed for epidural or intrathecal administration. Great care should be exercised in doing so and the patient should be informed of the risk undertaken. Particular attention should be paid to neurotoxicity of preparations.

Opioids are very commonly used. Hydrophilic drugs such as morphine are more likely to spread cephalad and to have systemic side-effects. Fentanyl and diamorphine are more commonly used. Good results with spinal opioids have been seen in patients with deep, constant, intractable somatic pain and in some neuropathic pains. There are many reports of successful treatment of pain by spinal administration of opioids including in the management of head and neck pain (by giving intrathecal morphine by a lumbar catheter).

Most often, opioids are used in combination with local anaesthetics.

Clonidine is effective as an addition in benign pain and is commonly used in malignant pain. It is of use when pain remains uncontrolled despite infusions of both opioid and local anaesthetic. It is effective through agonist actions at the $\alpha_2$ receptors of the dorsal horn, as well as increasing the effectiveness of the local anaesthetic and opioid. Claims have also been made for the effectiveness of baclofen.

## Technique

It has been suggested that intraspinal opioids should be trialled as to their efficacy and the patient's ability to tolerate the drug.

- Systemic opioids are reduced as opioids are introduced intrathecally or epidurally. An initial reduction in dose of at least 50% is recommended to minimize the risk of respiratory depression at the time of starting the infusion whilst still preventing a withdrawal syndrome. Amounts of fentanyl delivered from fentanyl patches must be reduced. As the half-life of a fentanyl patch is 17 hours, patch dose must be reduced several days before the commencement of intrathecal/epidural opiate infusion. Supplementary oral morphine must be given during the period when the fentanyl patches are being reduced and the patient awaits the procedure. Breakthrough doses of oral morphine may be needed after starting the infusion.
- Subcutaneous tunnelling of catheters is normally undertaken. It is suggested that this may have little role in the prevention of infection but protects against the catheter falling out. The externalization site of the tunnelled catheter is planned and marked, giving consideration to positional factors such as sites of waist bands and stomata. Catheters are tunnelled to the abdominal wall or the anterior chest wall.

- Local anaesthetic cream is applied preoperatively to the skin beneath which tunnelling will take place (marked by the operator).
- In the case of intrathecal lines prophylactic antibiotics are recommended by some workers.
- Both the epidural and intrathecal placement of lines involve percutaneous access through an introducer needle (e.g. Tuohy needle).
- Epidural catheters are placed in the lumbar, thoracic or cervical region dependent on the level of pain.
- Intrathecal catheters are placed in the lumbar region and if required they are directed cephalad.
- The catheter can be connected to an external infusion pump/syringe driver via further tubing and filter(s).
- Intrathecal catheters can be attached to a subcutaneous injection port, a subcutaneous reservoir, a patient-activated implanted reservoir system or a programmable implanted reservoir system.

# Problems and solutions

Some problems are due to the placement and use of the catheter and some are due to the drugs infused.

### Immediate

Local anaesthetic can cause hypotension, bradycardias, weakness or paralysis depending on the degree and height of sympathetic and motor block. Hypotension is treated by lying the patient flat, giving oxygen, intravenous fluids and where necessary vasopressors (ephedrine 3 mg intravenously (i.v.) increments, titrated against response). Bradycardia is treated with atropine increments of 0.3 mg i.v. Weakness affecting the muscles of respiration may necessitate ventilatory support. Opioids can cause respiratory depression or drowsiness. This can be treated by administering oxygen, naloxone 0.1 mg i.v. increments titrated against response and ventilatory support if necessary. Clonidine can cause hypotension and drowsiness.

### Early

Throughout the time of infusion bupivacaine can cause numbness and weakness. It may be inevitable. It has to be balanced against the need for local anaesthetic to provide analgesia. Pruritus, urinary retention and nausea and vomiting are side-effects of opioid infusions. They are usually transient but should be dealt with symptomatically as they occur. Pruritus can be treated with chlorpheniramine or naloxone.

### Late

Infection is a serious consequence of these techniques. It may be heralded by pyrexia, leukocytosis or neurological deficit. The intrathecal line allows sampling of CSF for microscopy, culture and sensitivity determination before its removal. The suspicion of an infected epidural line necessitates its removal for microscopy culture and antibiotic sensitivity of the tip.

Tachyphylaxis to both local anaesthetics and opioids may occur requiring increasing doses to achieve the same effect.

## Long-term management of lines

Once the patient is reasonably pain-free and without side-effects, the catheter can be managed within the community. Support and backup from the hospital is maintained. Protocols for management are drawn up and training is given to carers.

Intrathecal infusions controlled by syringe drivers are infused at a rate of 10 ml per 24 h. This necessitates daily changing of the syringe, a task which can be undertaken by community nursing staff or relatives. Strict asepsis must be observed. Reservoirs are replenished by hospital staff.

Epidural infusions may require larger volumes. These tend to be made up by hospital pharmacies under aseptic conditions. However, some units use the lower volumes associated with intrathecal use.

Regimes for the change of dressings for exteriorized lines must pay attention to infection control.

There should be daily inspection of exit sites or injection ports and daily recording of temperature, mobility and pain control.

## Further reading

Anderson PE, Cohen JI, Everts EC, Bedder MD, Burchiel KJ. Intrathecal narcotics for relief of pain from head and neck cancer. *Archives of Otolaryngology – Head and Neck Surgery*, 1991; **117:** 1277–80.

Onofrio BM, Yaksh TL. Long-term pain relief produced by intrathecal morphine infusion in 53 patients. *Journal of Neurosurgery*, 1990; **72:** 200–9.

Ventafridda V, Caraceni A, Sbanotto A. Cancer pain management in cancer pain. *Pain Reviews*, 1996; **3**(3): 153–79.

## Related topics of interest

Cancer – opioid drugs (p. 56); Cancer – other drugs (p. 60).

# CANCER – NERVE BLOCKS

*Andrew Severn*

The use of nerve blocks in cancer is less widespread than it has been. A better understanding of the use of morphine, less reluctance to use it for fear of dependence, and improvements in preparations of strong opioids, together with advances in psychological support, have resulted in an improvement in cancer symptom control. Nevertheless it was estimated, in 1989, that 10% of patients treated with morphine and similar drugs could not tolerate treatment, and a further 10% obtained no significant pain relief. Even with the introduction of alternative methods of opioid delivery, such as the spinal route, there remains a group of patients in whom a nerve block or nerve destruction procedure is appropriate. If successful, a total or substantial reduction in opioid dose and associated side-effects will be achieved. Nerve destruction is optimally carried out after assessment of the response to a local anaesthetic block: this step may be omitted if urgency or logistics dictates and the indications for nerve destruction are obvious. A local block may be of value, however, in that a response to a block may outlast the pharmacological action of the local anaesthetic, and chemical neurolysis may be postponed while repeat local anaesthetic procedures are carried out.

## Indications for nerve blocks

Pain should be localized or unilateral. Many patients with cancer have more than one pain: in this case, the pain site that is considered for nerve block should be considered to be a major problem in its own right. Visceral and somatic pain is more appropriately treated with nerve blocks than neuropathic pain. Opioids should have been tried and found wanting, either because of failure to achieve analgesia or because of unacceptable side-effects.

## Choice of method

Block of the sympathetic ganglia or chain is effective for the treatment of visceral pain, and has the specific advantage over blocks of the somatic nerve roots of preserving bladder and bowel control and normal sensation and movement. The choice lies between somatic blocks: intrathecal, epidural, peripheral nerves, interpleural, and blocks of the sympathetic ganglia or the nerves travelling through them.

## Specific techniques

*1. Intrathecal injections.* The intrathecal route for neurolysis is particularly useful for unilateral pain that is limited to the distribution of a few dermatomes. Major side-effects are sensory and motor loss, and loss of sphincter control. Intrathecal injections of neurolytic substances are used to destroy the dorsal (sensory) root of the spinal cord. The technique depends on the influence of gravity in distributing hypobaric and hyperbaric solutions of neurolytic substances through the cerebrospinal fluid, and the patient must be positioned accordingly. Furthermore, it is important to remember that the spinal cord is shorter than the spinal column and that for lesions of the lower thoracic roots, lumbar and sacral roots, the substance must be deposited at a more cephalad level than the exit foramen. Absolute alcohol is hypobaric, and the patient must be positioned with the target root uppermost. Phenol 5% in glycerol is a hyperbaric solution which requires the patient to lie on the side of the lesion.

Side-effects are prevented by a technique which allows the cooperation of the patient to report untoward motor loss. Alcohol causes pain in the appropriate dermatomal distribution, phenol results in a sensation of warmth. These observations allow the conscious patient's position to be altered slightly if, after injection, the target for the lesion has been missed. The block can be repeated, avoiding the risk of using too great a volume of neurolytic substance at any one time.

**2. Epidural injections.** A more widespread pain than those treated by intrathecal neurolysis can be treated with epidural neurolysis. The placement of an epidural catheter allows the adequacy of a local anaesthetic block to be evaluated, and allows phenol (in aqueous solution) to be added on an incremental basis, thus minimizing the risk of motor block.

**3. Interpleural injections.** Relief of the pain of tumour in the pleura and chest wall following the interpleural injection of phenol has been reported. The greater, lesser and least splanchnic nerves can be blocked via the interpleural route, as an alternative to coeliac plexus block.

**4. Peripheral nerve injections.** Many possible clinical indications exist, for example the use of intercostal phenol to treat the pain of an isolated rib metastasis. An alternative is the use of a catheter technique for local anaesthetic infusions. Chemical neurolysis of a nerve trunk will produce motor block and sensory block: in the context in which it is administered (i.e. terminally ill and bed-bound) this may be a small price to pay for comfort.

**5. Coeliac plexus block.** This remains a useful method for the relief of visceral pain associated with cancer of pancreas and stomach. The sympathetic block, in addition, results in an increase in gastric motility, with reduction in nausea and constipation. Following a successful coeliac plexus block, opioid consumption can be greatly reduced. Tumour may alter the anatomy of the region, making the block technically difficult. Neurolytic coeliac plexus block has been shown to be effective in 90% of patients with pancreatic or visceral cancer pain. The principal side-effect, and one which has to be considered, is the small (estimated at 1 in 600) risk of damage to the arterial supply of the spinal cord. In the context of the terminally ill or bed-bound patient this may well be an acceptable risk.

**6. Hypogastric plexus block.** This has an application for the treatment of pain from pelvic malignancy, although, as above, anatomy may be distorted by tumour.

**7. Ganglion impar block.** This ganglion is located deep to the coccyx and is a useful target for perineal lesions.

**8. Percutaneous anterolateral cordotomy.** This, probably underused technique, is appropriate for patients with unilateral pain. The technique involves the positioning of a radiofrequency lesioning probe in the spinothalamic tract at the level of the second cervical vertebra on the side opposite to the pain (the spinothalamic tract crosses the midline of the spinal cord just cephalad to the relevant dorsal horn). The procedure is performed with the patient lying supine and conscious, because the response to stimulation of the spinothalamic tract has to be noted. It is thus a major undertaking for the type of patient who could theoretically benefit most from it (chest wall pain from lung cancer or mesothelioma). Lesions of the tract corresponding to the lumbar and sacral dermatomes are easier than those for the cervical dermatomes. Immediate complications include respiratory depression from phrenic nerve damage; late complications include central neuropathic pain.

## Systematic review

Carr D, Eisenberg E, Chalmers TC. Neurolytic celiac plexus block for cancer pain – a meta analysis. *Proceedings of the 7th World Congress on Pain, Paris.* Seattle: IASP Press, 1993; 338.

## Related topics of interest

Cancer – intrathecal and epidural infusions (p. 49); Cancer – opioid drugs (p. 56); Neuropathic pain – an overview (p. 113); Therapy – nerve blocks: autonomic (p. 176); Therapy – nerve blocks: somatic and lesion techniques (p. 179); Therapy – neurosurgical techniques (p. 183).

# CANCER – OPIOID DRUGS

*Kate Grady*

Pain in advanced malignancy can usually be controlled by drugs. Opioids are the mainstay of treatment. They are used either alone or in combination with other analgesics. Pain may be uncontrolled despite the use of high-dose opioids.

## Principles of cancer pain treatment

**1.  *Multiplicity.*** Most cancer patients have more than one pain; 80% have at least two pains.

**2.  *Identification.*** Each pain must be clearly identified and treated separately.

**3.  *Effectiveness*** of treatment should be regularly reviewed.

**4.  *Efficacy.*** Not all pains are adequately treated by opioids. History, examination and investigation determine whether a pain is nociceptive and likely to respond to opioids or neuropathic and less likely to respond to opioid drugs and require antidepressants, anticonvulsants and other membrane-stabilizing drugs, etc. Other adjunctive treatments such as steroids may be needed. To ensure that a pain is still opioid sensitive, the breakthrough dose should be given (see later) and the patient reassessed for pain control after 20 min.

**5.  *Doses*** of opioid should be increased for as long as the patient remains in pain and that pain responds to the opioid.

**6.  *Side-effects.*** There must be close attention to and treatment of side-effects of opioid therapy (e.g. constipation).

## Choice of opioid drug

Guidance to the use of analgesics in cancer pain is given by the World Health Organization as the 'analgesic ladder'. There is, however, no scientific evidence to support the use of drugs in this way.

**1.  *Step 1.*** Non-opioid, for example, aspirin, paracetamol or nonsteroidal anti-inflammatory drug (NSAID) (may need to be substituted by a COXIB).

**2.  *Step 2.*** Weak opioid, for example, codeine, with or without non-opioid.

**3.  *Step 3.*** Strong opioid, for example, morphine, diamorphine or fentanyl, with or without non-opioid.

NSAIDs or COXIBs are the non-opioid of choice in steps 2 and 3 and are recommended in metastatic bone disease or soft tissue infiltration. Recommendations are ibuprofen 200–800 mg t.d.s. orally or diclofenac 50 mg t.d.s. orally.

## Choice of route

**1.  *Oral.*** The oral route is always preferable, unless precluded because of weakness, coma, dysphagia, vomiting or poor enteral absorption. Parenteral routes are not indicated simply because therapy is ineffective. Oral opioid treatment begins at step 2 of the analgesic ladder with codeine. Codeine is a prodrug of morphine. It is available in tablets of 30 and 60 mg and in various combinations with non-opioid analgesics. Most combined analgesics contain little codeine (8–10 mg). However Tylex, Kapake and Solpadol contain 30 mg of codeine plus 500 mg of paracetamol per tablet. Recommended dose of codeine is 30–60 mg 4-hourly. Codeine is very constipating. Laxatives must be prescribed. Pain uncontrolled by codeine should be treated at step 3.

The bioavailability of morphine may be as low as 20%. It is used in two main forms; one of immediate release and one of controlled or sustained release. Immediate-release morphine is available in both liquid and tablet form. It has rapid onset, peak effect within 30–90 min, and short duration, usually of 4 h. Controlled- or sustained-release morphine preparations have a different absorption profile. Modified release morphine tablets are prescribed on a 12-hourly basis and there are two newer preparations which are prescribed on a 24-hourly basis.

Assessment of requirements and adjustment of dose is accomplished using the immediate release preparation in the following way:

- Start oral morphine sulphate solution regularly (4-hourly). Dose suggested for the elderly or frail is 2.5 mg, in others 5–10 mg.
- Prescribe the same dose 2-hourly for breakthrough pain.
- If the regular dose is consistently inadequate or does not last 4 h, increase the 4-hourly dose by 30–50%.
- Once the patient has been pain free for a period of at least 24 h, the morphine taken in the last 24-h period should be totalled and prescribed in controlled release form, either as a twice daily dose of MST (total 24-h dose divided by two) or as a once daily dose of the 24-h preparations.
- One-sixth of the total daily dose of morphine should always be available as oral morphine sulphate solution for breakthrough pain.
- Patients should be warned that drowsiness, dizziness and nausea may occur but wear off within a few days. Antiemetics may be necessary. Constipation is the main persistent problem, so laxatives must be prescribed.

**2. Subcutaneous.** This route is used only when the oral route is not possible. Drugs are administered through a small cannula. Diamorphine is the drug of choice. (Hydromorphone is used outside Britain.) Its high solubility allows it to be dissolved in a very small volume of infusate. The potency of oral morphine to subcutaneous diamorphine is 3:1, so previous total daily oral morphine dose should be divided by three to give the 24-h subcutaneous diamorphine dose. When infusing a volume of 10 ml per 24 h, the subcutaneous site is effective for approximately 7 days. Breakthrough subcutaneous doses should be given at a sixth of the 24-h dose. The subcutaneous route is unsuitable where there is oedema, erythema, soreness, a tendency to sterile abscesses or a coagulopathy. Antiemetics and sedatives can be added to the infusate.

**3. Intravenous.** This may be necessary where subcutaneous infusions have failed.

**4. Rectal.** The oral preparations of immediate release morphine and MST tablets can be given in suppository form.

**5. Transdermal.** Fentanyl is delivered transdermally in the fentanyl patch. It provides equivalent pain control to morphine on the following basis:

| Oral morphine dose (mg per 24 h) | Fentanyl patch size ($\mu g\,h^{-1}$) |
|---|---|
| <135 | 25 |
| 135–224 | 50 |
| 225–314 | 75 |
| 315–404 | 100 |
| 405–494 | 125 |
| 495–584 | 150 |
| 585–674 | 175 |
| 675–764 | 200 |
| 765–854 | 225 |
| 855–944 | 250 |
| 945–1034 | 275 |
| 1035–1124 | 300 |

The 25 $\mu g\,h^{-1}$ patch is a suitable starting point with breakthrough oral morphine to allow further assessment and titration. Patches come in doses of 25, 50, 75 and 100 $\mu g\,h^{-1}$. It is anticipated that the means to deliver 12.5 $\mu g\,h^{-1}$ will become available. To increase the dose above 100 $\mu g\,h^{-1}$, combinations of patches are used. The fentanyl patch is effective and the patient does not need reminding of the need for medication. Each patch delivers the determined dose for 72 h before it requires renewal. In a small number of patients the patch needs to be renewed after 48 h. It can take 6–12 h to achieve analgesic levels in the plasma and levels continue to rise for up to 24 h. There is a slow fall in levels after the patch has been removed. After 17 h plasma levels are at 50%. These kinetics must be taken into consideration in changing from one form of opioid to another. Fentanyl patches have fewer side-effects than morphine, particularly constipation.

**6. Transmucosal.** Transmucosal fentanyl can be delivered by a lozenge with applicator. It has a licence in both malignant and non-malignant pain. It is intended for breakthrough pain in those on regular strong opioids. There may be a place for its use in incidental pain. It is intended to be used for no more than four episodes of breakthrough pain per 24 h. Should it be the case that satisfactory pain control is not achieved within this limit the dose of long-acting regular opioid should be increased. The lozenge is placed against the cheek and moved around. It is kept there for 15 min over which time the dose within the lozenge is absorbed. It can be removed from the mouth should side-effects occur during this time, and no more drug will be absorbed. This can be repeated 15 min later if pain control is not achieved but not again for this pain episode. Fentanyl lozenges are available in 200, 400, 600, 800, 1200 and 1600 $\mu g$ doses. If two doses have been required to treat an episode of pain or if that episode has not been controlled by two doses, the next increment in lozenge size should be used at the next episode. The patient should be carefully watched during the period of dose determination.

## Opioid rotation

Opioid rotation refers to a change to another opioid drug to achieve a better balance between analgesia and side-effects. If the usefulness of an opioid is thought of as a continuum, side effects also determine the place of that drug on the continuum. The pharmacological principles are as follows. Tolerance is said to occur when the dose of drug needs to be increased to give the same effect. It occurs to adverse effects and to analgesic effects. Cross tolerance refers to one drug causing tolerance to another. This can apply to both analgesic and side-effects. Tolerance can be less than complete. Switching to another opioid relies on cross tolerance for analgesia being less than cross tolerance for side-effects. The effect of changing drug is unpredictable because equianalgesic dose cannot be predicted as it depends on the degree of cross tolerance. Some would advocate an early switch as failure to respond well to one opioid does not means failure to respond to another.

Certain considerations must be made; there may be other causes of side effects than drug toxicity, and if pain is neuropathic it may be less responsive to opioids; consider other treatments for neuropathic pains. There are some who argue that the way to improve the side-effect–analgesia balance is to reduce the dose.

Methadone has been used in opioid rotation. It is a strong opioid whose action is enhanced by its NMDA antagonist effect.

## Tramadol

This interesting drug has a relatively low affinity for $\mu$ opioid receptors and its analgesia is only partially inhibited by naloxone, a selective $\mu$ opioid receptor antagonist. It has a second analgesic mechanism. It inhibits reuptake of serotonin and noradrenaline, thus modifying the transmission of pain impulses by enhancing serotonergic and noradrenergic pathways. The effects of the individual mechanisms in producing analgesia are modest, but in combination they are synergistic. This allows sparing of $\mu2$ opioid receptor side-effects. Tramadol is used as a transition between weak and strong opioids. It is said to be less constipating than other opioid drugs.

# Related topics of interest

Neuropathic pain – an overview (p. 117); Therapy – opioids in chronic pain (p. 189).

# CANCER – OTHER DRUGS

*Kate Grady*

## Non-opioid analgesics

Non-narcotic analgesics such as paracetamol, the salicylates, the nonsteroidal anti-inflammatory drugs (NSAIDs) and cyclooxygenase Type 2 inhibitors (COXIBs) are analgesics, anti-inflammatory treatments and antipyretics, with varying potencies for each of these actions.

The World Health Organization (WHO) recommends a non-narcotic analgesic for mild to moderate pain and recommends NSAIDs or COXIBs as a supplement to opioids for bone pain or soft tissue invasion. NSAIDs are of particular use when there is an inflammatory component to the pain. The use of an NSAID may allow reduction of the dosage of morphine. NSAIDs have a ceiling effect so recommended doses should not be exceeded.

Individual toxicity and patient response governs choice of NSAID. Toxicity is more likely in a cancer than a non-cancer patient because of co-existing disease. Patient response to each drug is variable and lack of response to one does not imply lack of response to others. For analgesic effect the drug should be tried for up to 2 weeks and if it is not successful another should be tried. Treatment should start with those of lowest toxicity. Ibuprofen has a low incidence of gastrointestinal side-effects (5–15%) and is a useful first choice at 200–400 mg t.d.s. Diclofenac has up to 25% side-effects at a dose of 50 mg t.d.s. Misoprostol protects against gastrointestinal side-effects and is available in combination with an NSAID. Meloxicam has a better side-effect profile because of its greater relative effect on the cyclooxygenase type 2 isozyme. Tenoxicam has been shown to be better tolerated than indomethacin. If side-effects persist despite these measures a COXIB such as celcoxib or rofecoxib may be advised.

Most NSAIDs are given orally but suppositories are available and ketorolac and diclofenac can be given parenterally. NSAID suppositories are used in the treatment of tenesmus.

## Corticosteroids

Pain with an inflammatory component can also be treated with corticosteroids. These reduce perineural oedema and are therefore used in central nervous system and spinal cord tumours. They are standard therapy for tumour-induced spinal cord compression. They are used in brachial or lumbosacral plexus invasion and can reverse early nerve compression. Pain from organ infiltration can benefit from corticosteroids. Pain from liver infiltration is improved by their effect in reducing capsular inflammation. They are given orally or intravenously. Suggested regimens are dexamethasone 2–24 mg per 24 h orally or a half to a third of this dose intravenously, or prednisolone 40–100 mg per 24 h orally. They should not be administered later than the early evening so sleep disturbance is avoided. Steroid enemas are used for the treatment of tenesmus.

Side-effects include adrenal axis suppression, sodium and water retention and hypertension, gastritis and peptic ulceration, reduced cell-mediated immunity and increased risk of infection, mood alteration and psychoses, hyperglycaemia, increased requirements for insulin and weight gain, myopathy and osteoporosis.

## Bisphosphonates

These are analogues of endogenous pyrophosphates which inhibit osteoclastic bone resorption. They are claimed to be effective in the treatment of cancer-associated hypercalcaemia. Increasingly they are used to treat intractable bone pain, particularly in myeloma. Pamidronate and clodrinate may be effective in reducing malignant bone pain. Clodrinate can be given orally and intravenously. Pamidronate must be given by intravenous infusion. Other bisphosphonates with therapeutic potential are aminohexane, risedronate and alendronate.

## Calcitonin

This also inhibits osteoclastic resorption of bone and is used effectively in the treatment of hypercalcaemia of malignancy. It has been said to be effective in the treatment of malignant bone pain at a dose of 100 IU b.d. subcutaneously.

## Nifedipine

Nifedipine at a dose of 5–10 mg t.d.s. is used for the treatment of painful oesophageal spasm and the relief of tenesmus.

## Hyoscine butlybromide

Colic due to malignant intestinal obstruction can be relieved by the smooth muscle relaxant hyoscine given 10–20 mg parenterally t.d.s. or 60–120 mg per 24 h by subcutaneous infusion.

## Oxybutinin

Painful bladder spasms may be relieved by oxybutinin. Patients should be warned of anticholinergic side-effects.

## Baclofen

The oral administration of baclofen, a γ-amino butyric acid (GABA) receptor agonist is used for the treatment of painful muscular spasms, 5 mg t.d.s. up to a maximum of 100 mg per day. It has also been used experimentally spinally. Unpleasant side-effects such as sedation, fatigue and hypotonia occur.

## Lignocaine

The subcutaneous infusion of lignocaine titrated against response with attention to toxic doses has been of effect in cancer pain.

## Nitrous oxide

A mixture of 50% nitrous oxide and 50% oxygen produces analgesia without loss of consciousness. It is self-administered using a demand valve. Excessive exposure by continuous use or frequent intermittent use causes megaloblastic anaemia from interference with vitamin $B_{12}$ synthesis. This might be considered an acceptable risk in a patient of short life expectancy.

### Chemotherapy/radiotherapy

Systematic review has confirmed the benefit of radiotherapy for bone metastases. In a large study 25% had complete pain relief at one month and 41% had at least 50% pain relief. Radiotherapy is the treatment of choice for bone metastases.

Specific cancer therapy may relieve pain if the cause of pain is direct tumour involvement. Careful evaluation of overall potential benefit has to be made before undertaking what can be unpleasant treatment.

## Systematic review

McQuay HJ, Collins SL, Carroll D, Moore RA. Radiotherapy for palliation of painful bone metastases. *The Cochrane Library*, Issue 4, 2000.

## Related topics of interest

Cancer – opioid drugs (p. 56); Neuropathic pain – an overview (p. 117).

# CHEST PAIN

*Kate Grady, Andrew Severn*

## Chronic refractory angina

Chronic refractory angina is a condition which is appropriately and successfully treated in the chronic pain clinic setting. The diagnosis is made where there is angina thought to be due to myocardial ischaemia due to advanced coronary disease despite optimal antianginal medication and where angioplasty or coronary artery bypass surgery have failed or are not feasible. The diagnosis should have been agreed by cardiologist, cardiothoracic surgeon and pain clinician. There should be regular cardiological review to ensure the patient has not developed new disease that needs revascularization and for supervision of antianginal medication. Assessment should ensure that the patient has in fact failed to respond and that poor compliance is not the cause. Similarly, obvious alternative diagnoses such as pain resulting from hyperacidity syndromes of the upper gastrointestinal tract need excluding before further management of the chest pain is contemplated: a trial of proton pump inhibitor should be considered. Pharmacological treatment should be rationalized in a multidisciplinary setting. A psychosocial history will help identify stressors and inappropriate beliefs, as well as helping to identify depression and anxiety.

Chronic refractory angina consumes a large amount of resources. A typical patient referred to a chronic refractory angina clinic has a severely curtailed quality of life and is demanding of medical resources. He or she is said to have a mean of 1.72 hospital admissions, 3.59 hospital outpatient visits, 6.5 GP surgery visits, 1.44 GP home visits and 0.55 attendances at A&E every year. The reported mean pain severity score is 6.6/10 and mean limitation of activity of 58%. 79.4% of patients with chronic refractory angina have been found to have symptoms of anxiety and 58% to be depressed. In addition it will be recognized that these patients have been failed by the traditional model of disease that has taught them and their carers that angina is a sign of imminent catastrophe! The pain clinician will appreciate that it is possible to change the way in which such fear is addressed. Angina that is refractory to medical treatment can be considered as a pain syndrome with much in common with other visceral pain syndromes. The authors of the National Refractory Angina Guideline make the following suggestions for management, recognizing that individual patients vary in their responsiveness for particular treatments. The guideline recommends a stepwise approach, in order of increasing invasiveness, risk of complications, and cost. Where effect and duration have been favourable there is a case to repeat treatments and possibly provide them on a regular basis as need arises e.g. temporary sympathetic blockade. The Guideline recommends:

### Counselling

Explanation of the management plan and lifestyle advice.

### Rehabilitation

This may reduce mortality and has been shown to reduce morbidity and symptom reporting and improve quality of life. Relaxation and stress management have both been shown to reduce angina.

## Multidisciplinary cognitive behavioural pain management programme

The most effective rehabilitation intervention has been shown to be exercise combined with psychological input.

## Transcutaneous electrical nerve stimulation

The mechanism of TENS in angina is unknown. It is used at continuous high frequency (70 Hz) for one hour three times a day and during angina attacks. Stronger stimulation may be needed during attacks. If it is to be used in a patient with a pacemaker the pacemaker may require reprogramming. The TENS machine should be trialled in the safety of the pacemaker clinic. The effect of TENS during an acute attack is usually immediate.

## Temporary sympathetic blockade

Angina involves the activation of afferent sympathetic pathways. Temporary interruption of sympathetic innervation can have an effect on pain. The effect and its duration are however not predictable.

In two thirds of patients sympathetic relay is at the level of the stellate and in one third it is at a low thoracic level. It was recognized as early as 1930 that infiltation of the stellate ganglion with local anaesthetic relieved angina and this has been substantiated by further studies. The injection of 15 ml of 0.5% bupivacaine to the left stellate ganglion can give lasting relief. Logically therefore, the stellate ganglion is the first choice for blockade, but the thoracic chain can be considered as a (more invasive) option in cases of failure to respond. Thoracic sympathetic blockade is performed by the injection of 15 ml of 0.5% bupivacaine at the paravertebral at T3/4 level on the left side or by thoracic epidural at the same level.

## Spinal cord stimulation

Spinal cord stimulation is used for prophylaxis or for the treatment of acute attacks. It has been shown to improve symptoms, quality of life, reduce number of ischaemic episodes, reduce glyceryl trinitrate consumption and reduce number of hospital admissions. It makes myocardial blood flow more homogenous thereby redistributing flow to areas which were previously ischaemic. An electrode is placed epidurally in C7/ T2 region under X-ray control. The level is adjusted to induce paraesthesia in the areas affected by the angina. It does not mask the pain of myocardial infarction and there is no increase in mortality rates in those who have a stimulator than in those who do not.

## Opioids

Opioids may be effective in relieving refractory angina. A careful trial is recommended. There may be a place for the intrathecal infusion of opioids.

## Interventional cardiology/minimally invasive techniques

Destructive sympathectomy and laser myocardial revascularization are procedures which may be tried in some centres.

# Non-cardiac chest pain

A substantial proportion of patients referred to cardiologists do not have underlying coronary artery disease, but are disabled by symptoms identical to angina. The condition cryptically referred to as 'Syndrome X' represents a group of such patients who demonstrate abnormalities of ECG on exercise testing but have normal coronary arteries on angiography. In such patients the cause of the pain has been variously described as due to microvascular occlusion, or due to alteration of the way in which the endothelial lining of blood vessels responds to local constrictor and dilator substances. These patients are amenable to the management strategies outlined above, with the added opportunity to address the symptoms as they would be in any other condition where the pain is not indicative of a life-threatening condition. As expected, the patient with non-cardiac chest pain or syndrome X presents with symptoms of psychological distress. A link between anxiety disorders and non-cardiac chest pain has been demonstrated, as has the high prevalence of panic disorder and depressive illness.

## Management

The same principles apply as to the management of refractory angina. Here, however, there is no potential life-threatening condition to which the symptoms may be attributed. Imipramine and clonidine have all been shown to reduce the frequency of episodes of chest pain, sertraline to reduce pain intensity. Cognitive behaviour therapy, particularly that which addresses the issues of catastrophizing and coping strategies, has been shown to be effective.

# Other chest pains

Pathology of the lungs and its associated structures can cause chronic pain. The pleuritic pain of interpleural adhesions from acute inflammatory disease can be treated with physiotherapy and nonsteroidal anti-inflammatory NSAID preparations.

An estimated 65% of adult cystic fibrosis presents with chest pain, the majority of these being in the last 6 months of life. The history usually reveals a worsening of pain over a two-year period. The pain is severe and usually in the anterior inferior part of the chest but may flit. It is exacerbated by coughing and breathing. It is a dull aching sensation felt to be within the tissue of the lungs and not in the chest wall. Whether it is a pre-terminal event or whether it seriously impedes expectoration and therefore precipitates death is unclear but the weight of opinion favours the latter. As such, this is a serious problem which kills. Formal quantitative sensory testing at one of the UK's leading neuropathic pain research centres has found the pain to be nociceptive.

It has been found to be unresponsive to paracetamol, ibuprofen, paracetamol and carbamazepine.

Opioids may have an adverse effect on pulmonary function and the constipation they cause results in problems in patients who require pancreatic supplementation for their malabsorption.

There are reports of the treatment of the pain by continuous epidural infusion but this is not without potential complications in this group of patients at risk of serious infections with atypical organisms. Capsaicin cream has been found to be partially effective in some but loses its usefulness as it causes an irritating cough in this group.

A pain similar in characteristic is seen in other chronic lung disease sufferers.

# Further reading

www.angina.org

## Related topics of interest

Assessment of chronic pain – psychosocial (p. 25); Depression and pain (p. 73); Therapy – nerve blocks: autonomic (p. 176); Therapy – opioids in chronic pain (p. 189); Therapy – spinal-cord and brain stimulation (p. 198); Therapy: TENS, acupuncture and laser stimulation (p. 206).

# COMPLEX REGIONAL PAIN SYNDROMES

*Andrew Severn, Kate Grady*

The complex regional pain syndromes (CRPS) comprise a variety of clinical presentations in which severe pain is associated with vasomotor changes and dysfunction in response to injury. Previously known as reflex sympathetic dystrophy and causalgia, the latter being a description of the presentation following specific nerve injury, they were reclassified in 1994 in an attempt to distance the syndromes from the implication that the sympathetic nervous system was always involved in the pathophysiology. However, the new taxonomy is by no means universally accepted, and references to the old taxonomy are regularly found in the literature. The syndromes also include conditions known as 'shoulder–hand syndrome', 'Sudek's atrophy' and 'algodystrophy'. The complex regional pain syndromes are neuropathic pain syndromes (type 2 is defined by the presence of nerve injury as the primary mechanism).

## Definitions and diagnostic criteria

### Complex regional pain syndrome type 1

Complex regional pain syndrome type 1 may follow an injury or event that causes immobilization. There are three mandatory criteria for diagnosis. These are:

1. Continuing pain, allodynia (painful response to a normally non-noxious stimulus) or hyperalgesia (heightened response to a painful stimulus) for which the pain is disproportionate to any inciting event.
2. Evidence at some time of oedema, changes in skin blood flow or abnormal sudomotor (sweating) activity in the region of pain.
3. Diagnosis is excluded by presence of conditions which would otherwise account for the pain and dysfunction.

### Complex regional pain syndrome type 2

1. Continuing pain, allodynia or hyperalgesia, following a nerve injury, not necessarily limited to the distribution of the nerve.
2. Evidence at some time of oedema, changes in skin blood flow or abnormal sudomotor activity in the region of pain.
3. Diagnosis is excluded by the presence of conditions which would otherwise account for the pain and dysfunction.

There is a good deal of heterogeneity in the presenting symptoms, but allodynia with draughts and clothing and extreme sensitivity to temperature changes are common. Type 2 often presents with allodynia combined with hypoaesthesia. Although the above criteria are sensitive, they are not specific, and a further diagnostic criteria is thus proposed.

Complex regional pain syndrome consists of pain that is disproportionate to any inciting event, and includes reports of at least one symptom in each of the following four categories:

- Sensory: reports of hyperaesthesia.
- Vasomotor: reports of temperature and/or skin colour change and/or skin colour asymmetry.
- Motor/trophic: reports of decreased range of motion and/or motor dysfunction (weakness, tremor, or dystonia) and/or trophic changes (hair, nail, skin).

Signs are reported in two or more of the following categories:

- Sensory: evidence of hyperalgesia to pin prick and/or allodynia.
- Vasomotor: evidence of temperature asymmetry and/or skin colour changes and/or asymmetry.
- Sudomotor/oedema: evidence of any of these and/or asymmetry.
- Motor/trophic: evidence of impairment, dysfunction or trophic changes.

## Pathophysiology

This is unknown. There are several theories.

*1. Autonomic nervous system.* Classically the inappropriate reaction of the sympathetic nervous system was implicated. This is a view that has been challenged. Autonomic involvement is often a feature but is inconstant and varies with time. Abnormalities of blood flow are demonstrated. This may be attributed to the sympathetic nervous system causing reflex vasomotor spasm and subsequent loss of vascular tone. However, gross limb blood flow is also related to the degree of muscle inactivity. It is thought that increased blood flow may cause excessive bone resorption to account for secondary osteoporotic changes. The degree of osteoporosis is often disproportionate to the degree of disuse. Neither definition (type 1 or 2) requires the role of the sympathetic nervous system in the maintenance of the symptoms, although it is tempting to assume that symptoms of temperature change, skin blood flow, and alterations in sweating are being mediated by the sympathetic nervous system. Blockade of the sympathetic system to the affected part has variable effects, and this may make for secondary differential diagnoses of 'sympathetically mediated' and 'sympathetic independent' pain.

*2. Inflammation.* CRPS has signs in common with acute inflammatory processes, namely changes in colour and temperature and the presence of swelling and pain. There is experimental evidence of disturbance of mitochondrial oxygenation. Oxygen extraction in the affected region has been shown to be impaired. Free radicals may be involved in what is possibly an untoward inflammatory reaction.

*3. Inactivity.* Immobilization or reluctance to use the affected limb severely exacerbates the syndrome and results in secondary changes such as localized osteoporosis, muscle contractures and muscle atrophy. Immobility reduces blood circulation: poor flow may account for the trophic changes seen in skin and nails.

**4. Central pain.** Although no clear mechanism has been defined, nor any clear link demonstrated, the development of CRPS after traumatic spinal cord injury and the presence of a similar syndrome in stroke victims suggest there could be a central mechanism.

**5. Psychological factors.** CRPS is a chronic condition and as expected, the patient's beliefs and prior experience of illness and injury will have bearing on the potential for recovery.

## Management

There are many theories as to how to treat CRPS. It is a progressive condition, since untreated it will progress to disability. It makes sense, therefore, to attempt to treat it as soon as the diagnosis is suspected. Management involves reducing the disability as well as the pain and the distress. Persuading the patient to move the affected limb is an important part of management.

Attempts to modify the sympathetic nervous system are commonly used in an attempt to provide analgesia. There are three strategies that have to be considered, intravenous sympathetic block, sympathetic ganglion block, and the use of drugs acting on the nervous system.

**1. Intravenous sympathetic block** using guanethidine in a limb isolated by a tourniquet is a commonly performed procedure in the pain clinic, is easy to perform and is often repeated. The evidence for its effectiveness as assessed by randomized controlled trials however, is far from convincing. A strong placebo effect has been noted, and it has even been suggested that the analgesic effect claimed is a consequence of ischaemia and pressure on the peripheral nerves from the tourniquet. Guanethidine is a drug with important cardiovascular side-effects if released into the systemic circulation prematurely (after deflation of the tourniquet). Thus there is a degree of controversy over the continued place of this procedure. In addition to guanethidine, various claims have been made for a variety of drugs, including bretylium, ketanserin and reserpine to be used in an isolated tourniquet technique. Local anaesthetic is usually injected with guanethidine to provide immediate pain relief and to prevent the pain of injection of the supposedly active drug. This will give a degree of analgesia that outlasts the tourniquet application and may allow a 'window of opportunity' for the patient to regain the ability to move the affected limb. Hence it is difficult to separate any claimed 'general' benefit of the procedure from the 'specific' benefit of the drug.

**2. Sympathetic ganglion block** is another frequently used procedure for CRPS of the limbs. Stellate ganglion block is used to block the sympathetic outflow of the upper thoracic ganglia that provide sympathetic fibres to the upper limb, and lumbar sympathetic block of the lumbar ganglia for the lower limb. The use of the latter has historically been associated with the use of open surgical techniques to destroy the lumbar sympathetic chain. More recently, thoracoscopic techniques have allowed the same procedure to be undertaken on the thoracic chain, and percutaneous chemical and radiofrequency lesioning techniques on the lumbar chain.

Tempting as it is to treat the patient who responds to a local anaesthetic block with a neurodestructive one, the long-term results are unconvincing. The procedures have not been formally evaluated with randomized controlled trials, and there are significant risks (neuritis of the genitofemoral nerve and a condition called post-sympathectomy pain) of the procedure that are difficult to predict and therefore difficult to avoid.

It is suggested that the very variable responses to sympathetic nerve destruction are the consequences of the very varied types of presentation and pathophysiology in CRPS. It is further suggested that progress in the future will depend on a reliable 'diagnostic test' for the involvement of the sympathetic nervous system in individual cases, allowing the clinician to avoid a potentially futile procedure if the pain is not relieved by the diagnostic test. To this end the intravenous phentolamine test is proposed. This requires the intravenous administration of phentolamine by infusion, 0.5–1.0 mg kg$^{-1}$ over 20 min. In practice, however, phentolamine testing requires the admission to hospital for a technique that involves an expensive drug, cardiovascular monitoring and cardiovascular risks similar to those of guanethidine intravenous block.

In summary, local anaesthetic blocks of the sympathetic nervous system may in some cases deliver short- to intermediate-term pain relief, but the ability to predict long-term success with nerve destruction is unproven. This may be because somatic pain relief is achieved in addition to sympathetic nerve block. The management of CRPS requires measures over and above an attempt to provide analgesia. It is vitally important that the patient is encouraged to regain normal function. This can be achieved under cover of repeated local anaesthetic blocks without recourse to an attempt to provide a 'permanent' solution.

The difficulty with assessing the effective treatments for CRPS lies with the varied presentations, the differing requirements of patients and the different expectations of patients and clinicians. For example, a randomized controlled trial that has as its criterion for success a 50% reduction in pain severity may fail to recognize as a positive effect a very substantial reduction of disability or an adequate level of pain relief that enables the patient to sleep properly. The continuing enthusiasm for sympathetic blocks by clinicians and patients despite poor 'high level' evidence may reflect the experience gained by many over many years. The placebo effect is, however, not to be forgotten.

**3.   Drug management.**   The action of certain antidepressants and anticonvulsants in neuropathic pain has been established, and so their use in CRPS, which by definition involves neuropathic pain mechanisms, is justified. Capsaicin cream has also been advocated. However, as with sympathetic block, it is important not to lose sight of the purpose of treatment, which is to persuade the patient to continue to move the limb, and in practice, any strategy which enables this to happen is acceptable.

In summary, the management of CRPS is a rehabilitation exercise, involving a stepwise progression through various physical and occupational therapy strategies.

These steps are as follows:
- Reactivation.
- Densitization.

Progressing to:
- Flexibility.
- Oedema control.
- Peripheral electrical stimulation.
- Isometric strengthening.
- Treatment of secondary myofascial pain.

Progressing to:
- Gentle increase in range of motion.
- Stress loading.
- Isotonic strengthening.
- Gentle aerobic conditioning.
- Postural normalization.

Progressing to:
- Ergonomics.
- Movement therapies.
- Normalization of use.
- Vocational and functional rehabilitation.

Oedema is managed by bandaging and lymph flow massage. Movement is optimized by scrubbing (for the upper limb, literally becoming able to scrub a floor on all fours with progressive force onto the scrubbing brush, or for the lower limb attaching the scrubbing brush to the foot) and other physiotherapy modalities such as extending range of movement, activity increase, strengthening and flexibility. Gait and posture correction and treatment of associated myofascial pains e.g. in the proximal joint, are also carried out by the physiotherapist. Other interventions, medications, injection techniques and cognitive behavioural therapy are introduced when the patient appears to be failing to make progress through the steps in the pathway.

# Further reading

Harden RN. A clinical approach to complex regional pain syndrome. *The Clinical Journal of Pain*, 2000; **16**(2): 26–32.
Jang W, Stanton-Hicks H (eds). *Reflex Sympathetic Dystrophy: a Re-appraisal*. Seattle: IASP Press, 1989.
Paice E. Fortnightly review: reflex sympathetic dystrophy. *British Medical Journal*, 1995; **310**: 1645–7.
Schott GD. Interrupting the sympathetic outflow in causalgia and reflex sympathetic dystrophy: a futile procedure for many patients. *British Medical Journal*, 1998; **316**: 792–3.

## Systematic review

Jadad AR, Carroll D, Glynn CJ, McQuay HJ. Intravenous regional sympathetic blockade for pain relief in reflex sympathetic dystrophy: a systematic review and a randomised double-blind crossover study. *Journal of Pain and Symptom Management*, 1995; **10**: 13–20.

## Related topics of interest

Neuropathic pain – an overview (p. 120); Sympathetic nervous system and pain (p. 153); Therapy – nerve blocks: autonomic (p. 176).

# DEPRESSION AND PAIN

*Kate Grady, Andrew Severn*

Pain and depression may occur concomitantly. Chronic pain may exacerbate depression. Chronic pain may be exacerbated by depression. The relative contribution and effect of each illness can be difficult to determine. Patients may not appreciate being questioned about symptoms of depression when they are consulting about symptoms of pain, but it is valuable to obtain a relevant history of symptoms of depression as a consequence of pain. In practice there is a risk that asking specific questions about depression may lead to a patient drawing a conclusion that the clinician is not taking the symptom of pain seriously. There is also a risk that important symptoms may be missed by the pain clinician. A multidisciplinary approach to patients who appear to be depressed may be of value. Conversely, expert opinion from a pain clinician about effective therapy may be valuable for the psychiatrist who otherwise may be tempted to explain the pain symptoms in terms of a depressive illness. There is a third reason for close liaison. This is that while antidepressant drugs are useful analgesics in a number of painful conditions, the most effective of these (tricyclics) have side-effects and are dangerous in cases of an overdose. In general terms, a clear diagnosis of depression requires proper and safe management of depression, even if this means antidepressant drugs such as serotonin specific re-uptake inhibitors (SSRI) which have limited analgesic effectiveness. An attempt to treat pain and depression simultaneously with one tricyclic drug may be possible, but the risk of attempted suicide through overdose should be discounted before this is done.

## Chronic pain exacerbating depression

An estimated 28% of patients attending pain clinics have a well defined affective illness. A greater number are dysphoric. Factors which worsen mood in a patient suffering from chronic pain are the inability to work, the futility of medical intervention and suggestions of their malingering. Patients become depressed during the course of a painful illness when they have not been depressed previously.

## Chronic pain exacerbated by depression

Approximately half of all depressed patients have pain. In a series of depressed women, atypical facial pain was the most common presenting symptom in 66%. In a smaller proportion of both sexes, tension headache was the most common presenting symptom of depression. Sites of pains which can be symptoms of depression are, in order of frequency, face, head, low back, limbs and abdomen. Characteristics of patients in whom pain may be a symptom of depression are low self-esteem, disturbed family circumstances, a personal history of psychological problems or a family history of psychiatric illness.

## Assessment of depressive symptoms in the chronic pain clinic

The additional presence of biological symptoms of depression such as loss of appetite and sleeplessness indicates that pain might be a symptom of depression. Self-rating questionnaires such as the Beck depression inventory, the Zung depression scale and the Hospital Anxiety and Depression scale are used. These tests do not constitute a full assessment, nor a psychiatric diagnostic process. They are quick, simple screening tools, allowing the subsequent interview to be focused.

### The need to distinguish depression from chronic pain

Unfortunately the common use of antidepressants and the presence of common features results in a blurring of distinctions in which it might be thought irrelevant to make an effort to diagnose depression in chronic pain patients. The diagnosis is important to make, however, if only because the doses of tricyclic antidepressant required for treatment of each condition are very different. Analgesic effect is independent of antidepressant effect. This is supported by evidence of an analgesic effect in non-depressed patients, by the early response of chronic pain to amitriptyline compared with the later response of depression and by the effectiveness of amitriptyline in the treatment of chronic pain at doses much lower than those required to treat depression. The principle of chronic pain management is to consider pain an illness in itself and not a symptom of other disease. This diagnosis is untenable if other diseases can account for the symptoms. If the disease in question is depression it must be identified and formally treated. Small doses of antidepressants, as used for pain management, may not be adequate. The use of invasive pain management techniques in a patient who is primarily depressed puts the patient at iatrogenic risk. Proper assessment protects against futile or potentially damaging medical intervention.

### Management of depressive symptoms in the chronic pain clinic

Support for the pain clinic may be provided by clinical psychologists or liaison psychiatrists. Psychologists are able to offer cognitive and behavioural treatments for depression in which negative thoughts and beliefs can be challenged and strategies developed for improving mood and psychological well being. Cognitive treatment may be ineffective if mood is very low, or severe biological symptoms are present, in which case medical management of depression is necessary. On the other hand, where there is a clear treatment for the pain clinic patient that can be used to treat the pain, mood may be seen to be improved as a result.

### Common mechanisms for pain and depression

A group of patients with pain without a physical explanation and not showing symptoms of depression was found to have an increased family history of depressive disorders. The pain responded to the use of antidepressants. Although at present distinctions are made in diagnosis and treatment, the interaction between pain and depression and the effectiveness of antidepressants in both illnesses suggests involvement of noradrenaline and serotonin in both. The role of common neurotransmitters suggests common pathology. This fact may be valuable when offering an explanation to the patient who is sceptical of the interest in depressive symptoms that the pain clinician is taking.

## Psychiatric nomenclature and chronic pain

The science of nomenclature of mental health problems allows experts from all professions in mental health to define syndromes using common diagnostic criteria. Some of these classifications have been used to describe conditions in which pain is experienced. The Diagnostic and Statistical Manual (DSM) classification of the American Psychiatric Association is one such system in common use. The fourth version of this system (known as DSM IV) recognizes a condition called 'pain disorder', or what is in this book referred to as 'the chronic pain syndrome', as a specific syndrome. Pain disorder, according to this classification is diagnosed when the following preconditions are met.

- Pain is the predominant presenting complaint.
- Pain causes significant distress or impairment in social, occupational or other important areas of functioning.
- Psychological factors are considered to play a significant role in the onset, severity, exacerbation or maintenance of the pain.
- The patient is not malingering.
- There is no better explanation, i.e. a mood, anxiety or depressive disorder.

DSM IV represents an advance on its predecessor, DSM III. DSM III described a condition called 'psychogenic pain'. This was defined as 'pain as an expression of psychopathology'. Although this recognized the importance of psychological factors in the pain experience, it implied an unhelpful dichotomy between physical and psychological causes, leading to an assumption that pain was either physical or 'in the mind'. This dichotomy is, unfortunately, too often reinforced when conventional medical thinking attempts to tackle a patient with the chronic pain syndrome, or the clinician cannot explain the symptoms and is looking for a 'way out' to refer the patient on to psychology services.

The WHO International Classification of Disease (ICD) version 10 is a parallel system to the DSM taxonomy. ICD refers to 'persistent somatoform pain disorder' as persistent distressing severe pain which cannot be fully explained by a physical disorder or physiological process, and 'somatization disorder', a condition associated with a poor prognosis and in which pain is one of many symptoms, such as breathlessness and abdominal bloating present over many years. Both diagnoses assume psychosocial causative factors.

The DSM IV taxonomy has taken the terms 'somatization disorder' and 'psychological factors affecting pain' out of the nomenclature in the belief that such classifications, as variants on the more comprehensive description 'pain disorder' suffer from the same disadvantages as the term psychogenic pain.

There are obvious advantages in the recognition of the condition called 'pain disorder' or 'chronic pain syndrome' into a mental health classification system. Significant amongst these is the realization that psychological factors may need to be addressed, with a chance for improvement. Responsibility for the management of the condition by professionals with a backgound in mental health problems is also recognized. For practical purposes we would recommend that the clinician who is not a specialist in mental health disorders satisfies himself or herself with the more comprehensive description of 'pain disorder', rather than trying to justify the term 'somatization' to colleagues or patients.

## Further reading

APA DSM IV TR Text: American Psychiatric Association, Washington DC, 2000.

## Related topics of interest

Assessment of chronic pain – psychosocial (p. 25); Therapy – antidepressants (p. 160); Therapy – psychological (p. 195).

# FACIAL PAIN

*Andrew Severn, Kate Grady*

The density of anatomical structures in the face, the significant representation of facial sensation within the cerebral cortex and the role of the face in personal and social interaction account for there being many causes and types of face pain. A variety of conditions present with facial pain. They vary from the clearly neuropathic with a well defined pathology, such as trigeminal neuralgia and post-herpetic neuralgia, through conditions in which there is a demonstrable pathophysiology, such as some presentations of temporomandibular pain and central post-stroke pain to those in which no pathology can be demonstrated, such as atypical facial pain. The importance of psychosocial factors cannot be underestimated: what the patient thinks about the significance of the pain has an important bearing on its perception, the degree of impairment and the way it is treated.

## Temporomandibular joint disease

This is taken to mean pain arising from the temporomandibular joint and the masticatory muscles. It can be classified into a disorder primarily of myofascial origin to be known as temporomandibular pain, and a disorder of the joint proper which will be referred to as internal derangement of the temporomandibular joint. It is appropriate to treat temporomandibular pain in the pain clinic. However the expertise of the faciomaxillary surgeon is often required initially to distinguish temporomandibular pain from pain due to internal derangement of the joint. Internal derangement of the temporomandibular joint should be managed by faciomaxillary surgeons. Temporomandibular joint disease occurs in a milder form equally in both sexes but those presenting for treatment (approximately 5–10% of the population) are female in a ratio of 8:1.

The validity of various theories such as occlusal derangement and bruxism remains unknown. Temporomandibular pain may be another form of musculoskeletal pain syndrome, including low back pain and the sufferer may experience the same psychological consequences as the sufferer from one of these syndromes. The importance of considering the psychosocial dimension should not be forgotten in coming to a diagnosis. The futility, and indeed danger, of adopting a purely biomedical view of the problem is the same – it leads to over investigation and unnecessary invasive treatment. An example of the dangers of the purely biomedical view is the treatment of pain with prosthetic implants into the temporomandibular joint which have subsequently been shown to be harmful.

Where the myofascial dysfunction is secondary to an occlusal problem, treatment of the underlying cause may benefit. The correction of occlusal abnormality resulting from an orthodontic problem or improperly filled tooth is necessary. Splinting devices are commonly used to this end. The difficulties in proving the benefit of such appliances are considerable. By 1995, 26 randomized controlled trials of 15 different splint devices had been identified. In the systematic review in which this was reported, the high placebo response rate was noted. A second systematic review reported a benefit of splint therapy in three controlled trials out of 14. As far as other symptoms are concerned, it is of interest that an occlusal splint was more effective for prevention of migraine than a placebo intraoral device which did not alter occlusion.

### Temporomandibular pain

This is intermittent pain of the ear, angle of the mandible or temple or can be less well localized. It can be bilateral. It is more intense in the morning or afternoon. It is exacerbated by movement or clenching. It is associated with joint noises and reduced range of joint movement. There is tenderness of the joint capsule and muscles of mastication and trigger points can often be elicited. It may run a prolonged course. Classically the pain is altered by the palpation of associated tender muscles and alleviated by the stretching of the muscle or the injection of local anaesthetic to the tender site.

### Treatment

In addition to the management of occlusal problems (see above), the following approaches have been reported of use in the treatment of muscle spasm. Injections to muscles of local anaesthetic alone are diagnostic but can be followed by the effective injection of steroid. Skeletal muscle relaxants such as baclofen at a dose of 5 mg t.d.s. are also used. Local muscle relaxation can be achieved with massage, heat and botulinum toxin. Claims are made also in respect of transcutaneous electrical nerve stimulation (TENS) and acupuncture. Generalized muscle relaxation can be achieved by relaxation therapies and biofeedback techniques. Cognitive strategies that recognize the importance of beliefs that the pain is disabling may be particularly valuable in this population. There is evidence from controlled studies that antidepressant drugs are effective.

### Internal derangement of the temporomandibular joint

This refers to distortion of the anatomy of the joint. Pain is exacerbated by jaw movement. There is swelling and tenderness of the joint and overlying muscles. Joint noises are common.

The cause is usually anterior displacement of the disc as a result of trauma, ligament laxity or changes in the fluid environment of the joint. The condition is not considered further here, since it is predominantly a surgical condition.

## Atypical facial pain

There is no single presentation of atypical facial pain. However pain tends to be present every day and lasts for most of the day. It can last from hours to months. It is a poorly localized, steady, deep burning or throbbing pain, and can migrate. It is unrelated to movement. It has no anatomically defined distribution and no associated physical signs. Sufferers are frequently depressed or demonstrate obsessive personality traits. It is most common in females over the age of 45 years.

### Treatment

It is most important to identify and treat the large contribution to pain from psychological, social and psychiatric factors. Medical treatment of depression may be necessary, including appropriate doses of antidepressants. Otherwise, the lower doses of antidepressants may be useful. Claims have been made for the combination of tricyclic antidepressant and phenothiazine, also for biofeedback and relaxation techniques, and transcutaneous nerve stimulation.

## Facial neuromata

Neuromata are common following facial trauma, particularly blow-out orbital fractures and Le Fort III fractures. They are frequently palpated at the site of exit of supraorbital, infraorbital and mental nerves. Diagnostic local anaesthetic nerve blocks can localize the site of pain, but there are obvious risks (of precipitating further neuropathic pain) if attempts to produce a more permanent nerve block are attempted.

## Systematic reviews

Antczak Bouckoms A, Marbach JJ, Glass EG, Glaros AG. Reaction Papers to Chapters 12 and 13. In: Sessle BJ, Bryant PS, Diohne RA (eds). *Temporomandibular Disorders and Related Pain Conditions*, Vol. 4. Seattle, IASP Press, pp. 237–45.

Forssell H *et al*. Occlusal treatments in temporomandibular disorders. *Pain*, 1999; **83**(3): 549–60.

Onghena P, Van Houdenhove B. Antidepressant induced analgesia in chronic non-malignant pain: a meta analysis of 39 placebo controlled studies. *Pain*, 1992; **49**(2): 205–19.

## Related topics of interest

Depression and pain (p. 73); Headache (p. 82); Neuralgia – trigeminal and glossopharyngeal (p. 107); Post-herpetic neuralgia (p. 133); Scars, neuromata, post-surgical pain (p. 142); Stroke (p. 150); Therapy – botulinum toxin (p. 166).

# GASTROINTESTINAL PAIN

*Andrew Severn*

This chapter considers painful disorders of the digestive tract including irritable bowel syndrome, burning mouth syndrome and non-ulcer dyspepsia. Differential diagnosis between the latter and non-cardiac chest pain (dealt with in a separate chapter) may be very difficult; both are usefully considered as visceral pain syndromes with common features.

## Irritable bowel syndrome

Irritable bowel syndrome (IBS) presents as crampy lower abdominal pain associated with either frequent loose stools or infrequent hard stools. Associated, distressing symptoms include bloating and a sensation of incomplete rectal emptying. Patients may complain of either diarrhoea or constipation.

The prolonged contractions of the colon which are suspected as being the major physiological alteration of IBS can be provoked by emotional factors. Stressful life events and a history of sexual abuse are worth noting as predisposing factors. IBS also occurs as a complication of infection of the gastrointestinal tract. The abnormal mechanoreceptor activation associated with a prolonged contraction may result in sensitization of primary afferents, and an exaggerated response to normally innocuous stimulation. This theory explains tenderness of the colon during palpation, and pain and spasm of bowel distension during sigmoidoscopy. The pain is therefore one of mechanical allodynia and hyperalgesia of viscera to non-painful and painful stimuli, respectively. The mechanism may be either one of primary afferent and dorsal horn sensitization or reduction of tonic supraspinal inhibition of autonomic afferent activity. It is possible that both mechanisms are acting, leading to a 'positive feedback' loop in which peripheral afferents become increasingly sensitized by removal of supraspinal inhibition. More severe cases of IBS complain of constant symptoms that are not relieved by the passage of stool.

## Non-cardiac chest pain and non-ulcer dyspepsia

Non-cardiac chest pain may account for up to 30% of admissions to coronary care units, and in view of the seriousness of the differential diagnosis of cardiac chest pain, may commit the physician to expensive, and risky, investigation (for example, coronary angiography). Abnormalities of oesophageal peristalsis and acid reflux may be responsible for pain in some cases, but there remains a group where neither of these account for the pain. This group of patients may have abnormalities of muscle regulation of oesophageal diameter associated with visceral hyperalgesia. Non-ulcer dyspepsia is therefore an analogous visceral pain syndrome to irritable bowel syndrome in the upper gastrointestinal tract.

## Burning mouth syndrome

Bilateral symptoms of burning affecting all areas of the mouth are the predominant features. The condition is more common in women and its appearance is typically between 50 and 60 years. Symptoms may be due to local pathology, notably candidal infection, xerostomia and lichen planus. Diabetic microangiopathy may also be responsible. Candidiasis may be a symptom of immunodeficiency or diabetes. Other associations such as changes in rheumatoid factor and antinuclear titres, and vitamin B and iron deficiency, have been noted but not explained. Subtypes of the clinical syndrome, as follows, reflect the many possible aetiologies, though the pain clinician may meet the patient after all reasonable attempts to find a cause have failed.

## Subtypes

- Type 1 worsens through the day, and may be associated with diabetes.
- Type 2 is present on awakening, persists through the day and may be associated with psychological problems.
- Type 3 runs a variable course, with days free from symptoms, a non-uniform distribution of symptoms, and may be associated with food allergy.

## Management

Psychological approaches, particularly methods involving relaxation, have a role in the management of all these conditions. Explanation of the cause of the condition may reassure the patient who is convinced of the serious nature of the condition, and seeks reassurance from repeated examination or endoscopy. The following account of therapies of the various syndromes is not exhaustive:

- *Hypnotherapy* has been shown to work in IBS.
- *Ispaghula husk and propantheline* has been shown to relieve symptoms of IBS and maintain remission.
- *Cognitive therapy* has been shown to reduce gastrointestinal symptoms in IBS and intensity of pain in burning mouth syndrome.
- *Loperamide* has been shown to reduce overall pain intensity, but at the expense of increased night pain.
- *Cromoglycate and antihistamines (ketanserin and H2 blockers)* have been claimed as effective drugs in the treatment of post-infectious IBS.
- *Antidepressants* have been claimed to be effective in both IBS and burning mouth syndrome.
- *B group vitamins* are claimed to be effective for burning mouth syndrome.
- *Smooth muscle relaxants* such as *nitroglycerin, hydralazine, nifedipine* and *diltiazem* have been described for treatment of non-cardiac chest pain. The mode of action is believed to be on the muscle of the oesophagus. That these drugs act also on the heart may lead to difficulties in diagnosis.

# Further reading

Mayer EA, Munakata J, Mertz H, Lembo T, Bernstein CN. Visceral hyperalgesia and irritable bowel syndrome. In: Gebhardt GF (ed.) *Visceral Pain, Progress in Pain Research and Management*, Vol. 5. Seattle: IASP Press, 1995; 429–68.

# Related topic of interest

Chest pain (p. 63).

# HEADACHE

*Andrew Severn, Kate Grady*

Headache which is not due to intracranial or systemic pathology is described as primary headache. Primary headaches are appropriately treated in the pain clinic, whereas secondary headaches require investigation. Diagnosis is made by history. Examination and investigations may be necessary to exclude secondary headache. Diagnostic criteria have been defined by the Headache Classification Committee of the International Headache Society.

## Migraine

Migraine is a primary headache. Diagnosis can be made from the history. However, investigation may be required to exclude headache of other aetiology.

### Pathophysiology

There are vascular and neural hypotheses. The ophthalmic division of the trigeminal nerve supplies painful structures within the head. Stimulation of the trigeminal ganglion releases a peptide from trigeminal neurones which innervate the cranial circulation. This peptide is called calcitonin gene-related peptide (CGRP). It is a powerful vasodilator. It is thought CGRP also causes neurogenic inflammation. Experimental work has been limited because of the absence of an animal model on which hypotheses and drugs can be tested. Agonists for a subtype of 5-hydroxytryptamine receptor known as 5HT1 agonists have been useful. The 5HT1 receptor has its own subpopulation of receptors, one of which, known as 5HT1δ, is involved in the mechanism of CGRP action.

### Diagnosis

Diagnostic criteria have been described by the Headache Classification Committee of the International Headache Society. Migraine is classified as *migraine without aura* and *migraine with aura* (*classical migraine*). The former is more common.

### Diagnostic criteria for migraine without aura

1. At least five attacks fulfilling criteria 2–4.
2. Headache lasts 4–72 h, untreated or unsuccessfully treated.
3. Headache has at least two of the following characteristics:
   - Unilateral location.
   - Pulsating quality.
   - Moderate or severe intensity (inhibits or prohibits daily activities).
   - Aggravation by walking up/down stairs, or similar routine physical activity.

4. During headache at least one of the following:
   - Nausea and/or vomiting.
   - Photophobia and phonophobia.

History, examination and/or investigation must exclude another disorder which could account for the headache. If such a disorder is present, diagnosis of migraine requires that attacks do not occur for the first time in close temporal relation to that disorder.

Premonitory symptoms can occur before an attack of migraine without aura. They usually consist of hyper- or hypoactivity, depression, craving for particular foods or repetitive yawning.

Aura is a complex of neurological symptoms which can initiate or accompany an attack. Symptoms may be localized to the cerebral cortex or brain stem. Typical aura are visual disturbances, sensory symptoms, weakness or dysphasia. Migraine aura can be unaccompanied by headache.

Migraine can be triggered by factors such as stress, withdrawal from caffeine, dietary factors such as the ingestion of chocolate, cheese, wines and seafood, and hormonal changes due to the menstrual cycle or hormonal medication. Stress and hormonal factors are each identified triggers in 60% of migraine sufferers. Dietary factors have been implicated in approximately 20%. Frequently there is a family history of migraine.

## Treatment

Management is by prevention of attacks and intermittent treatment of attacks. The choice between prophylactic therapy and the sole use of abortive treatments depends on the frequency, severity and impact of acute attacks.

## Prophylaxis

Drug therapy used for prevention aims to reduce the frequency of attacks by 50% and that attacks should be less severe when they do occur. The effect of the drug on the headache and its associated symptoms should be closely monitored. All drugs have side-effects and their benefits need to be accurately compared to their disadvantages.

Explanation and reassurance reduce the incidence and severity of attacks. Patients should be educated to avoid triggers where possible. Systematic review has been undertaken of the following therapies.

- *Calcium channel-blocking drugs* are effective in the prophylaxis of migraine. Flunarizine, nimodipine, verapamil, nifedipine and diltiazem are all equally as effective. A reduction in migraine frequency of approximately 50% can be expected after 2 months of treatment with any of these drugs. 'Systemically active' calcium blockers cause predominantly vascular and gastrointestinal problems, whilst 'cerebro-specific' calcium blockers cause behavioural and muscular side-effects.
- *Anticonvulsant drugs* have been shown to be effective. This suggests a neural mechanism for migraine. They are thought to work via γ-amino butyric acid (GABA) enhancement of inhibitory pathways.
- *β-Blockers* (for example, propranolol 80–240 mg daily in divided doses) are thought to have some activity at 5HT subreceptors. Propranolol has been shown to induce a 43% reduction in migraine headache activity. When improvements were assessed using further outcomes they were found to be 20% greater.

Propranolol 160 mg daily yielded a 44% reduction in migraine activity when daily headache recordings were used to assess outcome. With less conservative outcome measures there was a 65% reduction in migraine activity.

- *Relaxation and thermal biofeedback training* have been shown to yield an initial reduction in migraine headache activity of 43% which was estimated to be 20% greater at further assessment.
- *Pizotifen* is a 5HT antagonist that has been shown to confer a prophylactic benefit in patients who take sumatriptan for acute treatment of symptoms. Pizotifen does not alter the severity of migraine. Its proven effect therefore is one of reducing the use of sumatriptan. Its principal side-effect is weight gain.
- *Occlusal splinting devices* have been shown to reduce the frequency and duration of migraine. A trial design used a 'placebo' intraoral device that covered the palatal mucosa but did not alter the mechanics of occlusion.

## Treatment of attacks

Evidence from randomized controlled trials supports:

- *Sumatriptan.* This is a 5HT1$\delta$ agonist. Its major advantages are rapid onset and high efficacy. Given orally at a dose of 50 or 100 mg the attack is relieved in half to two thirds of patients. If the symptoms are not relieved a subsequent dose should not be taken. If symptoms are relieved but later recur a further dose can be taken, up to a maximum of 300 mg in 24 h. The subcutaneous injection of 6 mg relieves 88% of attacks. Headache settles in approximately 30 min. It should be used with caution in patients with a history of cardio-vascular disease.

In addition reports of success with the following have been made:

- *Paracetamol with metoclopramide.*
- *Nonsteroidal anti-inflammatory drugs (NSAIDs)* can be effective. They are given with antiemetics to treat a relatively mild attack. They have the advantage of being available in parenteral and suppository forms should nausea occur and preclude the oral route.
- *Biofeedback techniques, hypnosis and acupuncture* have also been used for the treatment of acute attacks. They are best used early.
- *Ergotamine* is given as a dose of 2 mg initially, repeated with 1 mg to a maximum of 5 mg. It is a powerful vasoconstrictor and should not be given to those with peripheral, cerebral or coronary vascular disease, nor to the pregnant patient or the known drug abuser.

# Cluster headache

This condition is otherwise known as migrainous neuralgia or Horton's syndrome.

## Diagnostic criteria

Pain is described as severe unilateral orbital, supraorbital or temporal pain lasting 15–180 min, every other day or up to eight times a day accompanied by at least one of the following, on the same side as the pain:

- Conjunctival injection.
- Lacrimation.
- Nasal congestion.
- Rhinorrhoea.
- Forehead and facial sweating.
- Miosis.
- Ptosis.
- Eyelid oedema.

History, examination and investigation must exclude another disorder which might account for the pain, or if such a disorder is present cluster headache should not occur for the first time in close temporal relation to the disorder. It is a disease found more commonly in men, in the fourth decade of life. Attacks occur in 'clusters' lasting 4–10 weeks. Most commonly they happen two or three times a day. Bouts of headaches often occur in early spring or early autumn. Clusters are interspersed by pain-free periods of months to years, but rarely more than two years.

Headaches usually last about 45 min. They can occur at any time of day but typically start soon after the onset of sleep. The pain is burning in character. Classically sufferers have deep nasolabial folds and *peau d'orange* skin changes. Precipitating factors include alcohol and altitude.

Cluster headache is thought to have a vascular mechanism.

## Management

Intranasal capsaicin has been shown to reduce headache severity. Sumatriptan has been shown to be effective. Other treatments for which benefit is claimed are:

- Abstinence from alcohol.
- Ergotamine 1–2 mg p.r. before the attack.
- Methysergide 2 mg t.d.s.
- Verapamil 40–80 mg t.d.s.
- Oxygen for 15 minutes during the attack.
- Sphenopalatine local anaesthetic block.
- Sphenopalatine ganglion radiofrequency lesions.
- Partial trigeminal nerve ablation.

# Tension headache

## Diagnostic criteria

The criteria for tension headache are the presence of at least ten previous headache episodes with frequency less than 180 headaches per year or 15 per month. The headache can last up to 7 days and should be accompanied by at least two of the following features:

- Pressing, tightening, non-pulsating.
- Mild or moderate.
- Bilateral.
- No aggravation by routine physical activity.

Nausea and vomiting are not features and photophobia and phonophobia should not be present together.

History, examination and investigation must exclude another disorder which might account for pain, or if such a disorder is present tension headache must not occur for the first time in close temporal relation to the disorder.

Headaches usually occur daily. There is a history of stress, and depression may coexist. It is more common in women. Overuse of analgesics may aggravate. Examination may reveal tender points.

## Management

Depression should be treated if present. Small doses of tricyclic antidepressants are also effective in those without clear signs of depression. The benefit of relaxation and cognitive strategies are claimed and nonsteroidal anti-inflammatory drugs (NSAIDs) are similarly said to be effective.

# Chronic paroxysmal hemicrania

This has the same features as cluster headache but attacks occur 15–20 times a day and last 3–15 minutes. It is more common in women and does not follow the onset of sleep.

## Treatment

Indomethacin 75–150 mg orally has been said to be effective.

# Cervicogenic headache

This is headache which originates in the structures in the neck. Pain from one or both sides of the neck radiates to the occiput, temples or frontal area. It is a dull pain, worse in the morning and exacerbated by movement or tension. Lateral flexion and rotational movements are restricted. Headache is often due to irritation of the C2 and C3 nerve roots and the greater occipital nerve.

## Management

Steroid injections to cervical facet joints give temporary relief in 60–70%. Benefits have also been claimed for greater occipital nerve blocks, transcutaneous electrical nerve stimulation (TENS), acupuncture and physiotherapy.

# Occipital neuralgia

This is a paroxysmal jabbing pain in the distribution of the greater or lesser occipital nerves. Aching can persist between paroxysms and there may be altered sensation. The affected nerve is tender to palpation.

The pain is eased temporarily by local anaesthetic block of the appropriate nerve. Subsequent injections of steroid are said to be effective.

# Analgesic headache

Large daily doses of aspirin, paracetamol or weak opioids taken for the treatment of headache can aggravate headache. The daily use of ergotamine for headache or sudden withdrawal from ergotamine induces headache. The withdrawal headache is thought to be due to vasodilatory counteracting mechanisms which have developed during the use of the drug but are left unopposed when the drug is withdrawn. Sumatriptan, used for the treatment of migraine causes the same problems.

## Management

Recommendations for prevention are:

- Analgesics should not be taken every day for the treatment of headaches.
- Ergotamine should not be taken more than 10 times a month.
- There should be restrictions on the use of all triptan type of drugs, such as sumatriptan, to approximately 10 times a month.
- Opioid drugs should not be used for the treatment of headache.

# Idiopathic stabbing headache

This is stabbing pain, predominantly in the distribution of the first division of the trigeminal nerve. It lasts for a fraction of a second. It occurs as a single stab or a series of stabs, at irregular intervals.

## Management

Indomethacin 25 mg t.d.s. is used to treat.

# Miscellaneous headaches

A number of primary headaches do not fit into these specific categories, such as those provoked by physical exertion, sexual activity, certain foods, very cold foods, coughing or restricting devices worn on the head. Avoidance of provoking factors should be advised where possible.

# Further reading

Classification Committee of the International Headache Society. Classification and diagnostic criteria for head disorders, cranial neuralgia and facial pain. *Cephalalgia*, 1988; **8** (suppl. 7): 1–96.

Connor HE. The aetiology of headache. *Pain Reviews*, 1994; **1**(2): 77–88.

Goadsby PJ, Olesen J. Fortnightly review: Diagnosis and management of migraine. *British Medical Journal*, 1996; **312**: 1279–83.

Olesen J. Analgesic headache. *British Medical Journal*, 1997; **310**: 479–80.

# Systematic reviews

Holroyd KA, Penzien DB. Pharmacological versus non-pharmacological prophylaxis of recurrent migraine headache: a meta-analytic review of clinical trials. *Pain*, 1990; **42**(1): 1–13.

Holroyd KA, Penzien DB, Cordingley GE. Propranolol in the management of recurrent migraine: a meta-analytic review. *Headache*, 1991; **31**(5): 333–40.

McQuay H, Carroll D, Jadad AR, Wiffen P, Moore A. Anticonvulsant drugs for management of pain: a systematic review. *British Medical Journal*, 1995; **311**: 1047–52.

Onghena P, Van Houdenhove B. Antidepressant induced analgesia in chronic non-malignant pain: a meta-analysis of 39 placebo controlled studies. *Pain*, 1992; **49**(2): 205–19.

Solomon GD. Comparative efficacy of calcium antagonist drugs in the prophylaxis of migraine. *Headache*, 1985; **25**(7): 368–71.

# Related topics of interest

Depression and pain (p. 73); Facial pain (p. 77); Neuralgia – trigeminal and glossopharyngeal (p. 107).

# IMMUNODEFICIENCY DISEASE AND PAIN

*Kate Grady*

## Acquired immune deficiency syndrome (AIDS)

The acquired immune deficiency syndrome is a painful disease. Not only is there a high incidence of patients reporting pain, but some two thirds of all patients describe constant pain interfering with their lives to a significant or severe degree. Many different pain syndromes are described, and patients present with more than one, said to be an average of three different pains. Not only is pain in AIDS inadequately treated, it threatens to pose a greater problem as survival rates improve.

Pain is due to disease or treatment. The pain profile is unique to the disease. There are significant psychological and social consequences of disease which have a bearing on the pain syndrome, complex medication of antiretroviral therapy and treatment and prophylaxis for opportunistic infections and cancers. Sufferers may be substance abusers which adds further complexity to the management of the condition. Patients are at increased risk of infection and neoplastic disorders and this should be borne in mind when providing symptomatic treatment.

Pain due to disease can be:

### 1. Gastrointestinal
- Oral and oesophageal candidiasis.
- Dental abscess.
- Aphthous ulceration.
- Mouth ulceration due to cytomegalovirus and herpes virus infection.
- Necrotizing gingivitis.
- Oesophageal ulceration.
- Gastrointestinal cramps associated with *Shigella*, *Salmonella* and *Campylobacter* infection.
- Small bowel obstruction and perforation, small bowel lymphoma.
- Cytomegalovirus colitis.
- Spontaneous peritonitis.
- Cholecystitis or cholangitis due to *Cryptosporidium* or cytomegalovirus infection.
- Proctitis and perianal abscess.

### 2. Neurological
- Brain tumour.
- Encephalitis.
- Aseptic meningitis.
- Cerebral toxoplasmosis.
- Cryptococcal meningitis.
- Painful symmetrical neuropathy due to direct action of HIV virus on peripheral nerves (affect approximately a quarter of patients).
- Cytomegalovirus infection of dorsal root ganglion.
- Demyelinating polyneuropathy.

### 3. Rheumatological

- Reiter's syndrome.
- Sacroiliitis.
- Polyarthralgia associated with mononucleosis.
- Psoriasis and psoriatic arthropathy.
- Reactive arthritis.
- Polymyositis.

### 4. Tumour

- Kaposi's sarcoma.

### 5. Pain due to treatment

- Pancreatitis is a consequence of retroviral therapy.
- Indinavir urolithiasis causing renal colic – requires hydration, narcotics and temporary cessation. If intervention is necessary endoscopic stent placement may be needed.
- Antivirals, antimicrobials and *Pneumocystis carinii* prophylaxis.
- Chemotherapy reaction, surgery procedures, bronchoscopies, biopsies.

The principles of pain assessment and management are not fundamentally different from those with cancer and justify the input of many professionals. Treatment may be pharmacological, anaesthetic, psychotherapeutic, and spiritual issues may have to be addressed also.

As far as analgesic management is concerned, the analgesic ladder is an accepted method of titrating drug potency to symptoms but due consideration must be given to the requirement for treatments for neuropathic pain and the use of psychotropic agents. Of interest is the requirement for opioids in patients with a prior history of opioid abuse. Patients may be tolerant of opioids, or anxious about using them. The principles of pain management in such patients include an acceptance that opioids may be appropriate, that there may be a potential for abuse, but more importantly that adequate pain relief can not be witheld because of fears of potential abuse.

## Further reading

Larue F, Fontaine A, Colleau SM. Underestimation and undertreatment of pain in HIV disease: multi-centre study. *British Medical Journal*, 1997; **314**: 23–9.

O'Neil W, Sherrard JS. Pain in human immunodeficiency disease: a review. *Pain*, 1993; **54**: 3–14.

## Related topics of interest

Cancer – opioid drugs (p. 56); Therapy – opioids in chronic pain (p. 189).

# MULTIPLE SCLEROSIS

*Kate Grady*

Multiple sclerosis (MS) is a progressive disease. It is characterized by initial destruction of myelin and eventually axons and cell bodies. It can affect any part of the central nervous system (CNS). It is well established that MS is a painful condition. There are varying reports of the incidence of pain such as:

- 40% of MS patients are never pain-free;
- 64% report pain at some time of their disease;
- 48% have more than one pain;
- 32% of pain sufferers with MS rate pain amongst the most severe symptom of their disease;
- Prevalence of pain for the preceding month has been quoted at 53%.

Pain can be:

- Disease related;
- Disability related.

There should be routine assessment for pain in MS patients with attention given to each pain.

## Disease-related pain

Pain related to the disease tends to occur when the disease is well established, although 23% have pain at the time of onset of the disease. The proportion of time in pain increases with disease severity, but pain intensity does not increase with disease severity. The number of people in pain increases with disease duration. Of those in pain 44% have difficulty sleeping and 34% have difficulty with personal relationships. Pain results in poorer mental health and increased social handicap. Pain from MS is predominant in females at a ratio higher than the female predominance of MS itself. The incidence of pain due to MS increases with age.

Pain peculiar to MS sufferers is of two types.

### Persistent neuropathic pain

Persistent pain occurs in an estimated 17–66% of MS patients. Lesions anywhere in the CNS may be the cause of pain but lesions of the spinal cord, lower brain stem and periventricular areas of the forebrain are more likely to be the cause. Although the demyelinating process of MS causes conduction block, secondary reorganization of membrane electrical properties occurs causing hyperexcitability and pain.

Pain tends to be extensive. It frequently affects the legs but can occur in more than one area. It is often described as burning and demonstrates allodynia and hyperalgesia. Visceral afferents can affect pain.

### Intermittent pain

Intermittent pain is due to:
- *Spasms and tonic seizures* – more likely to occur if spasticity is uncontrolled.
- *Tightening painful sensations of the extremities.*

- *Trigeminal and glossopharyngeal neuralgias* – these may be caused by demyelination of the brain stem. Trigeminal neuralgia occurs in up to 5% of MS sufferers. It differs from primary trigeminal neuralgia in that there is a constant background of pain with superimposed spasms of pain, typical of classical trigeminal neuralgia, it occurs in a younger population, and is more likely to be bilateral. Of those with bilateral trigeminal neuralgia, 18% have MS.
- *L'Hermitte's sign.* This sign refers to the occurrence of an electrical sensation passing down the back to the legs on flexion of the neck. It is reported at some time in up to 25% of MS patients. It is related to disease involving the dorsal columns and cervical nerve roots. It is not always painful.
- *Abdominal pain.* This is thought to be neuropathic and occurs in 2% of sufferers.
- *In a girdle or radicular distribution* occurring acutely in the absence of obvious nerve compression. This may be due to demyelination of root entry zones and is perceived as burning pain.

# Disability-related pain

## Musculoskeletal pains

These are caused by postural and musculoskeletal abnormalities arising from paresis, spasms, discoordination and immobility.

Low back pain increases with disease duration. Approximately 39% have low back pain.

## Peripheral neuropathic pains

Nerve compression secondary to musculoskeletal deformities can cause neuropathic pain.

Although depressive symptoms and cognitive disturbances are recognized in MS sufferers the incidence of such symptoms does not differ between MS sufferers with pain and MS sufferers without pain.

# Treatments

Each pain must be dealt with separately albeit that treatment of more than one pain may be achieved by a single pharmacological tool. Attention must be given to associated symptoms of psychological distress.

The general principles of treatment of neuropathic pain are applied to the persistent pain, the neuralgias, optic neuritis, sometimes to the abdominal pain and to neuropathic pain arising from disability.

Treatment should start with the tricyclic antidepressants with anticonvulsants as second line of treatment. Gabapentin and lemotrigne have been reported to be of use.

Treatment of *pain due to spasm, tonic seizures and spasticity* has been the subject of many controlled trials. Unfortunately, few trials used a reliable and validated measurement of spasticity such as the Ashworth Scoring System. Gabapentin proved effective over a 48-hour period and was then chosen and used for long-term therapy in one trial. Other drugs used in trials, but described in a systematic review as lacking in adequate methods for measuring spasticity include baclofen, dantrolene, tizanidine, botulinum toxin, vigabatrin, prazepam and threonine. Reports claim the benefit of carbamazepine, epidural clonidine, baclofen (both orally and intrathecally) and spinal cord stimulation. There are reports as to the effectiveness of cannabis lasting several hours after administration. Reports of mexilitine effectiveness are tempered by suspicion that paralysis may appear to worsen. There may be a place for implanted spinal infusion catheters for the delivery of drugs such as baclofen in selected patients.

## Trigeminal neuralgia

Although surgical treatment for primary trigeminal neuralgia in the operation of microvascular decompression is effective, this is not so for trigeminal neuralgia due to MS, where the characteristic pathology of primary trigeminal neuralgia is absent. Trigeminal neuralgia secondary to MS is shown to be best treated with anticonvulsant drugs, the most popular choice being carbamezepine. Five out of six patients treated with topiramate 25 mg b.d. increasing by 50 mg per week up to a maximum of 200 mg b.d. had complete relief. There are also reports of the success of percutaneous retrogasserian glycerol rhizotomy (reports of 38–88% complete relief ) and radiofrequency lesioning of the ganglion. Glossopharyngeal neuralgia associated with MS responds to carbamezepine.

1. *L'Hermitte's sign* pain is said to respond to weak electromagnetic fields but this is not a widely available treatment.

2. *Abdominal pain* may be treated by sympathetic blockade using local anaesthetic alone. This technique may provide pain relief beyond the pharmacological duration of the local anaesthetic.

## Musculoskeletal pain

Physiotherapy assessment is valuable for determining the relative contribution of the musculoskeletal system to the presentation of pain, and for the supply of appropriate appliances and local treatments. Standard analgesics, including anti-inflammatory drugs where appropriate may be of value also. Transcutaneous electrical nerve stimulation (TENS) and acupuncture may be of value if the cutaneous sensation is preserved, but may be ineffective, even poorly tolerated, if the nerve pathways from primary afferent large diameter fibres are affected by the disease process. As in any case presenting with low back pain, sinister pathology and surgically operable lesions must be excluded. Treatment may be difficult as provoking factors are likely to persist. Radicular pain can be treated by drugs effective for neuropathic pain. Epidural steroids may be considered, but there is a potential medicolegal hazard in using a drug without a product licence on a central nervous system suffering from an unpredictable and progressive disease.

## Further reading

Clifford DB, Trotter JL. Pain in multiple sclerosis. *Archives of Neurology*, 1984; **41:** 1270–2.

Kassirer MR, Osterberg DH. Pain in chronic multiple sclerosis. *Journal of Pain and Symptom Management*, 1987; **2**(2): 95–7.

Stenager E, Knudsen L, Jensen K. Acute and chronic pain syndromes in multiple sclerosis. *Acta Neurologica Scandinavica*, 1991; **84:** 197–200.

## Systematic review

McQuay H, Carroll D, Jadad AR, Wiffen P, Moore A. Anticonvulsant drugs for the management of pain: a systematic review. *British Medical Journal*, 1995; **311:** 1047–52.

Shakespeare DT, Young CA, Boggild M. Antispasticity treatments for multiple sclerosis. *The Cochrane Library*, Issue 4, 2000. Oxford: Update software.

## Related topics of interest

Back pain – injections (p. 35); Facial pain (p. 77); Therapy – anticonvulsants (p. 158); Therapy – antidepressants (p. 160); Therapy – Cannabinoids (p. 169).

# MUSCULOSKELETAL PAIN SYNDROMES

*Barrie Tait, Andrew Severn*

Joint pain is a presenting feature of many conditions outside the scope of this textbook. Where pain is associated with synovitis and progressive articular cartilage destruction, there is a clear requirement that treatment of the disease process is a key part of the management of pain and the reduction of disability. Pain is to a large extent nociceptive, with the additional factor that chronic nociceptive states induce a permanent state of hyperexcitability of the central nervous system, and chronically painful conditions cause secondary changes in mental well-being and function. The specific management of conditions in which inflammation is part of the disease process will not be discussed here. The reader is referred to rheumatology textbooks for details of the management of rheumatoid arthritis, ankylosing spondylitis, polymyalgia rheumatica and gout. It is worth noting, however, that the disease process of rheumatoid arthritis can be affected by the central nervous system. Thus, rheumatoid arthritis is not observed in joints of a limb affected by a stroke. Palindromic arthritis, a type of rheumatoid arthritis with flitting joint pains and inflammation has been claimed to respond to block of the sympathetic system.

The musculoskeletal pain syndromes to be discussed here include the syndromes termed fibromyalgia and myofascial pain syndrome, together with conditions associated with a painful shoulder. In these conditions the pain and disability may be considered part of a pain syndrome rather than the result of a progressive nociceptive process. Non-specific low back pain has many features in common with these syndromes.

## Fibromyalgia and myofascial pain

The syndromes have as common features symptoms of regional or widespread tenderness. The validity of using separate diagnostic criteria, implying distinct pathology, is questionable. There is a risk that, in focusing on specific pain complaints in the search for symptom relief, the strategy of reducing disability will be ignored. Some authorities have considered the concept of a condition such as fibromyalgia so unhelpful that they have suggested an alternative name, the 'irritable everything syndrome'. One interpretation is that musculoskeletal pain syndromes are overlapping syndromes, variants of muscle pains that otherwise healthy individuals suffer.

### Definitions

Given the limitations above, attempts to define individual syndromes are as follows:

*1.  Fibromyalgia.*   Widespread pain: this means bilateral pain, and pain below and above the waist, in addition to neck or back pain.

Pain on digital palpation, using a standard force (4 kg) in 11 of 18 possible sites. The sites are described bilaterally in the following positions and are by convention referred to as 'tender points':

- Suboccipital muscle insertions.
- Anterior aspect of transverse process C5–C7.
- Midpoint of upper border of trapezius.
- On the medial border of the spine of the scapula.
- Costochondral junction of second rib.
- Distal to the lateral epicondyle.
- The upper outer quadrant of the buttock.
- Posterior to the greater trochanter of femur.
- Medial aspect of lower end of femur.

Three-quarters of patients with tenderness in 11 or more of these sites complain of fatigue, sleep disturbance or morning stiffness, and over half complain of headache or pain 'all over'. Sleep disturbance, as described in association with tender points and widespread pain has particular electrophysiological features.

**2.    *Myofascial pain syndrome.*** There is no requirement for the pain to be widespread. Areas where pain is experienced on palpation are, by convention, called trigger points. Trigger points are specific for particular muscles. Pain is experienced in a characteristic regional distribution when trigger points are stimulated. Trigger points are described as occurring within one area of a taut band of muscle fibres, which if snapped in a transverse direction is associated with a local twitch response.

## Pathophysiology

It has not proved possible to identify a peripheral source of abnormal nociceptor activity in these conditions, although attractive theories concerning metabolic origins for areas of taut muscle fibres abound. Histological and biochemical studies have so far failed to prove these theories. Lowering of threshold to electrical stimulation is not restricted to tender or trigger points identified clinically, but is part of a widespread disorder, and therefore one of central processing.

## Management

The following symptoms should alert to the possibility of serious or systemic disease for example inflammatory arthritis and temporal arteritis:

- Morning stiffness.
- Tenderness over the superficial temporal artery.
- Joint tenderness or swelling.

Regional pain may be perceived in the referred dermatomal distribution of visceral pathology, persisting after the visceral problem has ceased to be a medical problem. Where there is history of trauma, consideration should be given to the spectrum of disorders known as 'complex regional pain syndrome'. Trigger points can be treated with precise needling of the point. The nature of any substance injected is less important than the mechanical disruption of the taut band that is achieved by needling. Local anaesthetic, steroids and neurolytic substances have their advocates. Longitudinal stretching of taut bands can be performed by the therapist or the patient. However, symptom control is no more important than advice about exercise and posture to prevent recurrence.

The evidence for any particular treatment of fibromyalgia syndrome is difficult to assess. The diversity of symptoms and the number of potential outcome measurements that could be made mean that it is difficult to interpret the data from randomized controlled trials. There is no consensus for the use of particular outcome measures: one of the more popular measures, a simple physician-rated scale of global improvement, demonstrates improvement in several drug trials. A systematic review commented that the use of amitryptiline is supported by two out of four randomized controlled trials, using measures of patient-reported pain, physician-reported pain and patient overall (global) assessment, and two out of three trials assessing patients' sleep.

Formal psychosocial and functional assessment with appropriate cognitive/behavioural approaches may be required for patients who do not respond to the measures outlined above.

# Frozen shoulder

There is no accepted definition of frozen shoulder and there is no well-defined pathophysiological process. It may be due to scarring in the capsule surrounding the joint. Symptoms are pain and severe restriction of active and passive movement particularly external rotation. It affects 2% of adults usually in the 40–60 years age group. In 20% it subsequently develops in the other shoulder. It is described as having three phases:

- Initial phase is the development of pain over 2–9 months. Pain is worse at night.
- Pain subsides over the subsequent 4–12 months but stiffness and restriction of movement persist.
- The third phase lasts 5–24 months and during this time pain and stiffness resolve.

The course can however take much longer and even when symptoms have resolved there can be some limitation in movement. Important conditions such as tendonitis, tears of rotator cuff, arthritis, joint infection, locked posterior dislocation of the glenohumeral joint and systemic disorders must be excluded. Tears of the cuff and tendonitis cause pain and restriction of active movement but not of passive movement as does frozen shoulder. Investigation of these disease entities includes full blood count, erythrocyte sedimentation rate, rheumatoid factor and shoulder X-ray.

## Treatments

The authors of a systematic review concluded that the effects of treatment were small.

- *Non-steroidal anti-inflammatory drugs (NSAIDs).* A systematic review showed these drugs were better than placebo in relieving pain and improving function when used for a few weeks.
- *Corticosteroid injections.* Steroids are injected into the subacromial bursa and into the joint itself. The injection of 20 mg methylprednisolone in 0.5 ml of 1% lignocaine three times weekly has been shown to improve mobility over the first four weeks but not in two weeks beyond that. A comparison between 40 mg methylprednisolone with lignocaine or lignocaine alone has failed to show a

difference. Three injections of triamcinolone 40 mg over 6 weeks has been shown to be superior to physiotherapy in improving pain and disability.

- *Oral steroids* Ten mg prednisolone daily for 4 weeks followed by 5 mg daily for 2 weeks with movement exercises has been shown to be superior to exercise alone for the first few weeks but there is no difference at 5 months.
- *Physiotherapy* includes mobilization, ultrasound, laser, TENS, magnet treatment, cold therapy and exercises. It has been shown that exercise is superior to analgesia alone in improving movement and superior to intra-articular triamcinolone alone in improving pain and mobility.
- *Suprascapular nerve block* of 10 ml of 0.5% bupivacaine three times at 7 day intervals alone has been shown to produce reduction in pain 2 weeks after the injection.
- *Manipulation under anaesthesia* has been reported to bring about good improvement but there was no statistical analysis of the data in the trial.

## Systematic review

Green S, Buchbinder R, Glazier R, Forbes A. Interventions for shoulder pain (Cochrane review). *The Cochrane Library*, Issue 4, 2000, Oxford Update software.

Van der Windt DAWM, van der Heidjen GJMG, Scholten RJPM, Koes BW, Bouter LM. The efficacy of NSAIDs for shoulder complaints. A systematic review. *Journal of Clinical Epidemiology*, 1995; **48:** 691–704.

White KP, Harth M. An analytical review of 24 controlled trials for fibromyalgia syndrome. *Pain*, 1996; **64:** 211–17.

## Related topics of interest

Back pain – medical management (p. 29); Nociceptive pain – an overview (p. 117); Osteoarthritis (p. 121); Therapy – anti-inflammatory drugs (p. 162); Therapy – physical (p. 193).

# NECK PAIN

*Andrew Severn, Paul Eldridge*

Painful neck syndromes are a heterogeneous group of conditions in which many mechanisms may be acting, but in which attention has in particular been directed to two sites of possible pathology: these are the cervical discs and the facet joints. The use of diagnostic nerve blocks has allowed the relative contribution of each site to persistent pain to be determined. In addition to pain arising from joints or discs, there may be muscular pain and pain due to irritation or compression of the cervical or brachial plexus. Secondary hyperalgesia may complicate the clinical presentation and make the precise diagnosis of origin of pain very difficult. Furthermore, other conditions, such as the musculoskeletal pain syndromes and headache syndromes include neck pain amongst the symptoms. It is also important not to miss aspects of the condition that might have a psychosocial dimension.

## Cervical spine trauma and pain

Pain after cervical spine trauma is frequently seen as a consequence of a rear-end impact in a road traffic impact, where it is colloquially termed a 'whiplash' injury. It is estimated that some 20% of victims subjected to this mechanism of injury will develop symptoms. It appears to be more common in women.

### Pathophysiology

Acute muscle injury occurs and may be the cause of pain in the acute stages, but other significant injuries include cervical spine fracture, prevertebral haematoma and damage to the recurrent laryngeal nerve. Muscle spasm of the scalene muscles may be responsible for some of the neurological symptoms referred to the arms, including a functional thoracic outlet syndrome. Primary brain injury may also occur, and be responsible for a psychological disturbance in the chronic syndrome. There is a substantial body of opinion which believes that the primary pathological mechanism is an arthritic process in the cervical facet joint, with pain referred to dermatomes according to the level of injury.

Other mechanisms which have been suggested to be of importance in the symptom complex include:

- Damage to the sympathetic autonomic supply to the head.
- The cilio-spinal reflex (neck pain associated with ipsilateral pupillary dilatation).
- Altered proprioceptive information from abnormally active cervical efferents leading to disordered vestibular function.
- Reflex inhibition of muscles supplied by segmental levels which receive nociceptive inputs.

### Clinical presentation

The principal symptom is of pain in the back of the neck which is worsened by movement and may radiate to the head, shoulder, arm or interscapular region. The headache is suboccipital and radiates anteriorly. There are other symptoms which may mimic signs of a general somatoform pain disorder, but in this particular instance may have a nociceptive or neuropathic cause:

- Visual disturbance.
- Vestibular difficulties.
- Weakness and heaviness of the arms.
- Paraesthesiae of medial side of hand.
- Dysphagia/hoarseness.
- Auditory disturbance.

## Investigation

No investigation is needed to confirm the clinical diagnosis of whiplash injury, but the circumstances of the injury usually require that a lateral X-ray of the cervical spine is taken. Fractures of the cervical spine can occur without impact, and specialized views e.g. laminar and pedicle views with computed tomography (CT) examination may be needed.

Diagnostic block of the medial branch of the cervical dorsal ramus has suggested that over 50% of patients have pain arising from cervical facet joints.

## Treatment

There have been many approaches claimed to treat the acute symptoms and those of the chronic syndrome. The use of selective local anaesthetic block followed, if successful, by radiofrequency lesion of the sensory supply to the cervical facet joint, the medial branch of the primary ramus of the appropriate cervical root has been shown to be effective. Pain relief of greater than six months is reported. In contrast, intra-articular injections of the facet joints may provide short-term pain relief of diagnostic significance, but the addition of steroid to the local anaesthetic did not confer an advantage in one study.

Other treatments that have been tried and reported include:

- Local heat, soft collar and physiotherapy.
- Occipital nerve blocks, diagnostic and neurolytic.
- Cervical epidural injections.
- Sympathetic nerve blocks.

Attempts to prevent the onset of a chronic condition have been unsuccessful: spontaneous remission of symptoms after 3 months is unlikely. The link between ongoing litigation and persistence of symptoms is debatable: in one study 45% continued to have symptoms two years after settling of claims. The assumption that patients with neck pain after cervical spine trauma in a road accident are exaggerating symptoms for financial gain is an oversimplification that causes unnecessary suffering in patients. It is important to recognize that psychosocial distress is a common accompaniment of many painful conditions, and that the manifestation of this distress is contingent on factors such as the way in which society treats victims of accidents, the attitude of employers and the benefits system. Thus patients with neck pain following whiplash injury may demonstrate illness behaviour in the same way as patients with other painful conditions, and measures to deal with the behaviour may be part of the treatment. It should not mean that the diagnosis of psychosocial distress should in any way prejudice the outcome of legal proceedings.

# Cervical spondylosis

## Pathophysiology

This diagnosis describes the changes caused by narrowing of the cervical nerve root foramina by bone or cartilage from osteophytes and hypertrophic facet joints. Such a definition supposes that the nerves in the foramina undergo pathological change, and it is to be expected that the sufferer would present with radicular symptoms.

## Clinical presentation

The pain syndromes associated with cervical root involvement are well described and consistent, although symptoms in adjacent nerve root territory may compound the clinical picture. Pain in the distribution of the nerve tends not to involve the hand, although paraesthesiae may be experienced. Upper cervical root compression is experienced as pain over the occiput and mastoid area. Nerve root compression is aggravated by axial loading, and by coughing, sneezing, jugular vein compression and extension of the neck.

## Investigation

The diagnosis of cervical spondylosis is a radiological one. As with other chronically painful conditions of the spine, there is a poor correlation between the radiological appearance and the symptoms.

## Management

The contribution of the cervical facet joints to the overall pain syndrome can be assessed by specific diagnostic nerve blocks (medial branch of dorsal primary ramus) or intra-articular steroid injection. Cervical epidural steroid and paravertebral injections may be used for pain with radicular features. It is noteworthy that there has been a recent case report of a high tetraplegia following a properly conducted cervical paravertebral steroid injection.

Electromagnetic field therapy has compared well with placebo for the reduction of pain. Otherwise there is a hierarchy of procedures of increasing difficulty using radiofrequency nerve lesioning techniques that can be used for neck pain with and without nerve root involvement. These are described as:

- Facet joint denervation.
- Stellate ganglion lesion.
- Cervical dorsal root ganglion lesion.
- Cervical disc lesion.

The greater occipital nerve, a continuation of the dorsal ramus of the second cervical nerve, can be blocked just lateral to the external occipital protuberance. Many conditions in which neck pain is experienced are more properly described as one of the musculoskeletal syndromes: cervical spondylosis simply being a convenient clinical description of a radiological observation. As with any other painful musculoskeletal condition, the contribution of psychological factors, such as those engendering a fear of movement should be addressed.

# Cervical disc disease

As with lumbar disc disease it may be completely asymptomatic and be found on imaging. It is common for cervical films to show evidence of osteophyte and loss of disc height with increasing age. A combination of disc prolapse and osteophyte formation produces the clinical picture which may be a combination of radicular effects and myelopathy. Disc prolapse, with or without the addition of root compression due to osteophyte presents as a combination of neck pain and brachalgia. The neck pain may radiate into the interscapular area and also to the occiput. Brachalgia is in the distribution of the appropriate nerve root and may be accompanied by sensory and motor deficits. In 90% of cases the lesion will be at C5/6 or C6/7.

Myelopathy may occur in association with the features described above or in its own right. Typical is the development of a spastic gait; in addition there may be problems with use of the hands indicating that a quadriparesis is present. Another syndrome, usually typical of compression at C3/4 is 'numb clumsy hands'. Not all cases progress and it is estimated that as many as 40% can be managed conservatively.

## Diagnosis

Diagnosis is almost universally by MR imaging, which has all but replaced myelography. If there is signal increase in the spinal cord prior to decompression, in cases of myelopathy, the prognosis is poorer for recovery.

## Medical treatment

Medical treatment follows the same principles outlined in the discussion above on cervical spondylosis. Disc abnormalities, as demonstrated with magnetic resonance imaging, may be associated with other abnormalities. While a surgical assessment is important to rule out progressively disabling disease, many patients with symptomatic cervical discs can be managed with medical means. Cervical epidural steroids and paravertebral steroid injections may be used, and attention to other features, such as the facet joints may be valuable.

## Surgical treatment

For single level disease approach is from anterior; there is disagreement as to whether or not fusion should be performed at the time of disc excision. However, if a simple discectomy is performed then fusion will ultimately result though taking a longer time than if a bone graft is used, and with the possibility of a small amount of kyphosis. Traditional approach is by Cloward's procedure or Smith Robertson in which some of the vertebral body is removed across the disc space. Iliac crest graft is used to 'plug' the defect and aid fusion after the disc and osteophytic compression of the nerve root has been cleared. Relief of brachalgia in 90% of cases is reported. The same procedure is used in cases of myelopathy though a difficulty arises when multiple levels are involved. Cloward's procedure can be carried out at multiple levels but increasingly surgeons may perform a trench vertebrectomy, with grafting and plate fixation. If levels are multiple then historically posterior laminectomy has been the procedure of choice. For myelopathy the goal is to arrest deterioration though improvement may also occur.

## Further reading

Barnsley L, Lord S, Bogduk N. Whiplash injury. *Pain*, 1994; **58**: 283–307.
Ferrari R, Russell AS. Epidemiology of whiplash: an international dilemma. *Annals of the Rheumatic Diseases*, 1999; **58**: 1–5.

## Systematic reviews

Gross AR, Aker PD, Goldsmith CH, Pelos P. Physical medicine modalities for mechanical neck disorders. *The Cochrane Library*, Issue 4, 2000.

## Related topics of interest

Assessment of chronic pain – psychosocial (p. 25); Back pain – injections (p. 35); Musculoskeletal pain syndromes (p. 95); Therapy – nerve blocks: somatic and lesion techniques (p. 179).

# NEURALGIA AND PERIPHERAL NEUROPATHY

*Kate Grady*

A neuropathy refers to dysfunction in a nerve secondary to nerve damage. It can affect a single nerve (a mononeuropathy) or many nerves (a polyneuropathy). It may or may not be painful. A bilateral symmetrical neuropathy is usually of systemic cause. A painful mononeuropathy is often referred to as a neuralgia.

## Pathophysiology

Localized or systemic damage and disease can cause demyelination of nerves and less frequently axonal degeneration. Consequently there is a barrage of afferent impulses to the dorsal horn of the spinal cord. This results in central sensitization. Ectopic impulse generation occurs both at the sites of damage and from associated degeneration in the dorsal root ganglion and the spinal cord. Damaged axons become hypersensitive to mechanical and chemical stimuli. Different nerves are affected by different types of damage. Damage may be non-selective, may affect only large fibres or may affect only small fibres. The type of fibre affected has bearing on the symptoms. Although the presence of pain is not related to fibre size alone damage to smaller fibres more often tends to cause pain. Rapid degeneration is more likely to cause painful neuropathy. Ephaptic transmission (neural cross-talk) causes the provocation of pain by normally non-painful stimuli such as touch.

# Painful polyneuropathies

Painful polyneuropathies tend to have a systemic cause. They are most frequently due to toxic agents, metabolic disorders or vitamin deficiencies. They present various patterns of sensory, motor or autonomic deficit. The lower limbs are usually affected, with sensory symptoms prevailing over motor symptoms. The more common ones are described below.

## Diabetic neuropathy

This is caused by small fibre damage. Sensorimotor deficiency and autonomic instability occur. Pain is tingling, burning, stabbing or shooting. Pain may also be due to peripheral vascular disease, joint disease or the development of ulcers secondary to reduced sensation.

## Alcoholic neuropathy

This is compounded by concurrent dietary insufficiencies. Non-selective damage occurs causing a sensory and motor deficit. Pain is burning with tenderness of the feet and legs.

### Nutritional deficiency neuropathy

Vitamin B1 and niacin deficiencies cause peripheral neuropathy. An associated condition, burning feet syndrome, does not necessarily have the clinical signs of peripheral neuropathy but responds to dietary enhancement of the B vitamins.

### Neuropathy due to drugs

Neuropathy from isoniazid therapy is characterized by spontaneous pain and paraesthesiae, worse at night. It is due to large fibre damage. Other toxic agents include certain chemotherapy agents, arsenic and mercury.

Painful peripheral neuropathies also occur in hypothyroidism, myeloma, amyloid, Fabry's disease, acquired immunodeficiency syndrome (AIDS) and as a dominantly inherited form. The peripheral neuropathy of chronic renal failure is often painless but there may be troublesome paraesthesiae or restless legs.

## Painful mononeuropathies and neuralgias

Damage to single nerves results from direct trauma, invasion by tumour, past surgery and compression or entrapment.

Examples include carpal tunnel syndrome, cranial, facial and intercostal neuralgias, radicular pain and *meralgia paraesthetica* (lateral cutaneous nerve of thigh). Within the distribution of the nerve there is pain with associated numbness, hyperpathia or allodynia. Sometimes this presentation, and the associated disability is more widespread than the distribution of the nerve itself, and is described as a Complex Regional Pain Syndrome (type 2).

### Management

Suspicion of an undiagnosed or undertreated systemic disease warrants investigation and treatment outside the pain clinic. Dietary neuropathies improve with supplements. Myeloma neuropathy can improve with antineoplastic treatments. Similarly entrapment neuropathies may warrant the opinion of a surgeon.

The treatments specifically for pain follow similar principles for both poly- and mononeuropathies and neuralgias. However extensive areas of involvement in the polyneuropathies often make the use of topical treatments impractical.

- *Physiotherapy.* Exercise and use is said to be important to maintain central input from non-nociceptor afferents.
- *Nerve blocks.* A sympathetic component to the pain may be sought. Sympathetically maintained pain is diagnosed as a response to blockade of the sympathetic nervous system, either by block of a ganglion or the intravenous use of guanethidine. The use of such techniques or drugs to maintain analgesia in response to an initial positive response is controversial, and is not well supported by evidence. Nor does the initial success with a local anaesthetic sympathetic block guarantee long-term success with a neurolytic agent. The difficulty in management of neuropathies with these techniques is that the response is variable and unpredictable. In respect of pain that does not respond to sympathetic block, a local anaesthetic somatic block may be of value to reduce the pain in the short term, but somatic block with a nerve lesioning technique

offers no realistic long-term solution: indeed it may result in a deafferentation pain that is worse than prior to treatment. Somatic blocks may however have a place as part of a strategy of encouraging movement about a painful joint affected by the pain, and it is an attractive, though unproven idea, that local anaesthetic blocks allow the central nervous system to restore the normal physiology that existed before sensitization. Somatic block may also be undertaken with a combination of local anaesthetic and steroid – the logic here being to reduce oedema that may be contributing to the condition.

- *Topical treatments.* Systematic review has demonstrated that capsaicin 0.075% cream applied four times daily for 4–8 weeks is effective in the treatment of painful diabetic neuropathy. Other topical treatments include the infiltration of the affected nerve with steroid, glycerol injections or the topical application of local anaesthetic or creams. The application of TENS to stimulate nerves proximal to the areas of damage has been reported to be of value.

- *Antidepressants.* Systematic review has demonstrated the value of tricyclic antidepressants (TCA) for many neuropathic pains. Paroxitene, a serotonin specific reuptake inhibitor (SSRI) has been shown to be effective in painful diabetic neuropathy.

- *Anticonvulsants.* Systematic review has demonstrated that anticonvulsants are effective for trigeminal neuralgia and diabetic neuropathy. Gabapentin is the only drug specifically licensed for neuropathic pain of any description, but by no means the only drug shown to be effective, and the choice of gabapentin over carbamazepine is determined more by side-effect profile than efficacy.

## Systematic reviews

Collins SL, Moore RA, McQuay HJ, Wiffen P. Antidepressants and anticonvulsants for diabetic neuropathy and post herpetic neuralgia: a quantitative systematic review. *Journal of Pain and Symptom Management*, 2000; **20**(6): 449–58.

McQuay H, Carroll D, Jadad AR, Wiffen P, Moore A. Anticonvulsant drugs for management of pain: a systematic review. *British Medical Journal*, 1995; **311**: 1047–52.

McQuay HJ, Tramer M, Nye BA, Carroll D, Wiffen PJ, Moore RA. Systematic review of antidepressants in neuropathic pain. *Pain*, 1996; **68**: 217–27.

Zhang WY, Li Wan Po A. The effectiveness of topically applied capsaicin: a meta-analysis. *European Journal of Clinical Pharmacology*, 1994; **46**: 517–22.

## Related topics of interest

Complex regional pain syndromes (p. 67); Neuralgia – trigeminal and glossopharyngeal (p. 107); Neuropathic pain – an overview (p. 113); Nociceptive pain – an overview (p. 117); Scars, neuromata, post-surgical pain (p. 142);Therapy – anticonvulsants (p. 158); Therapy – antidepressants (p. 160); Therapy – nerve blocks: autonomic (p. 176).

# NEURALGIA – TRIGEMINAL AND GLOSSOPHARYNGEAL

*Paul Eldridge*

There are now recognized a number of neurovascular compression syndromes of which trigeminal neuralgia (TGN) is the best understood. Since this is the one most relevant to a pain practice it is discussed in more detail; of the other conditions glossopharyngeal neuralgia is worth mentioning.

## Trigeminal neuralgia

This is an unusual example of a neuropathic pain that may be amenable to surgical correction in which a potential cause is removed.

### Incidence and prevalence

The incidence is estimated to be 50/million/year and the prevalence at 155/100 000. It is of increasing frequency with age.

### Pathophysiology

In approximately 90% of cases a vessel, usually an artery, is found in contact with the trigeminal nerve at the root entry zone as it exits the pons. Sometimes this contact may groove the nerve. It is not clear how such contacts cause TGN, but sensory malfunction can be detected in the laboratory, as can abnormalities of the trigeminal somatosensory evoked response. Normalization of neurophysiology and sensation occurs following microvascular decompression, and the usual outcome from the procedure is instantaneous pain relief. All of these observations argue that the neurovascular contact or compression is important in the causation of the condition. It has also been proposed that spontaneous discharges occur within a hyperexcitable trigeminal ganglion – the equivalent of the dorsal root ganglion in the spine where similar behaviour has been observed following spinal injury. The combination of this factor with the effect of neurovascular contact at the root entry zone, perhaps causing demyelination, or a multiple sclerosis (MS) plaque in the trigeminal system results in the paroxysmal nature of the pain and its intermittent course. A total of 2–4% of cases of MS suffer trigeminal neuralgia whilst 5% of cases of trigeminal neuralgia are in association with MS.

### Clinical features

The clinical features of the condition have been defined by both the International Association for the Study of Pain and by the International Headache Society. The pain should be unilateral in the distribution of one or more branches of the trigeminal nerve. The pain is sharp and stabbing in quality coming in paroxysms. There are trigger points which are usually circumoral hence the pain is provoked by chewing, talking and wind on the face. The pain is intermittent in nature with remissions lasting several weeks or months. A response to treatment with carbamazepine is typical and it is refractory to conventional analgesics including anti-inflammatory agents and opioids. In the majority of cases the pain involves the second or third divisions, and only relatively rarely is the pain purely in the first division.

## Signs

In classical teaching there are no signs, though a decreased corneal reflex may occur. Therefore any neurological deficit found on bedside testing should raise the suspicion of a structural lesion, or of idiopathic trigeminal neuropathy. However, quantitative sensory testing carried out in laboratory conditions will reveal subtle sensory deficits undetectable clinically.

## Differential diagnosis

From a spectrum of other facial pain and headache syndromes. Conditions referred for clarification of diagnosis include atypical facial pain, cluster headache, painful trigeminal neuropathy and temporo-mandibular joint dysfunction. Perhaps surprisingly dental pain is rarely seen in the pain clinic though a large number of patients have first passed through a dental practice. Although classically described as trigeminal neuralgia, pain from structural lesions such as the extremely rare trigeminal schwanoma or lesions in the region of the cavernous sinus is different being continuous, progressive and associated with neurological deficit.

## Investigations

No specific test exists for this condition. However MR techniques are now available which detect the presence or absence of neurovascular contact at the root entry zone with a sensitivity of 100% and specificity of 96% validated in a series of 55 cases. The same studies reveal that neurovascular contact may be found in almost 10% of controls so the MRI findings should not be relied on to prove the diagnosis but used to influence the choice of treatment. Some attempts have been made to demonstrate pre-operatively neurophysiological abnormalities, particularly far-field evoked potentials, but these have not proven to be either sufficiently sensitive or specific.

## Management

The natural history of the condition is for the severity of attacks to worsen and for the periods of remission to shorten. Symptomatically the syndrome may evolve from its typical form to a variant in which there is a constant background burning element to the pain, in addition to the classical features. There may also be the development of subtle sensory impairment.

*1. Drug management.* The drug of first choice is carbamazepine. Whilst effective, treatment with this drug is not without problems. It is difficult to estimate accurately the numbers of patients who 'fail' medical treatment. Reasons for failure are idiosyncratic reactions to carbamazepine (rash being typical) and dose-related problems. At high dose – to which the patient is driven by the severity of the pain – there may be ataxia and severe drowsiness. However the cognitive impairment produced by the drug 'in normal usage' is underestimated and may be the principal reason why some sources have found failure rates with carbamazepine reaching 75% of cases treated. Analysis of studies concludes that the number needed to treat for effective pain relief ( > 50% compared to control) is 2.6 and the number needed to harm is 3.4. One long-term study exists where either loss of effect or intolerance occurred in over one half of patients over ten years.

Alternatives that have been reported to be effective include lamotrigine, phenytoin, sodium valproate, gabapentin and baclofen. All have been reported to be effective in combination though there is no published study comparing monotherapy and polytherapy.

Withdrawal of medication should be gradual because of the risk of provoking a seizure; however although this can occur it is rare. Patients often stop their medication quite rapidly of their own volition when entering a period of remission without experiencing this complication.

Sodium valproate and phenytoin find application in the acute situation as they can be given intravenously.

*2. Foramen ovale or Gasserian ganglion methods of nerve block.* The trigeminal ganglion is approached via the foramen ovale. Fluoroscopic imaging is required. Peripheral lesions of the divisions of the trigeminal nerve using alcohol or nerve avulsion will not be discussed in detail, save to say that there is a high rate of pain recurrence and late deafferentation pain.

*3. Radiofrequency lesioning.* A needle is introduced via the foramen ovale; electrical stimulation performed to confirm correct placement of the needle by inducing paraesthesiae in that area of the face that the trigeminal neuralgia is occurring. The patient is then anaesthetized and a thermo-coagulation performed (60–90°C for approximately 45 seconds). Although originally suggested that heat preferentially destroyed selectively thin pain fibres, using formal sensory testing it was found that all fibres are affected approximately equally. It is difficult to target the ophthalmic division, and this runs the risk of corneal anaesthesia. A further risk is of masseter weakness and for this reason the technique is rarely performed bilaterally.

Over 90% will experience immediate relief of pain; however with time there is a gradual recurrence rate. Recurrence rates vary with series, and range from as poor as 25% pain free at two years to up to 80% pain free, and the recurrence rate seems to be related to the technique. If deep hypoalgesia is produced during the procedure, essentially by creating a larger lesion, the recurrence rate is lower. Unfortunately the larger the lesion the greater the risk of creating dysaesthesias, and the feared complication of *anaesthesia dolorosa*. In series with low pain recurrence rates the higher dysaesthesia rate is found; 25% of cases exhibit dysaesthesia regarded by the patient as unpleasant but tolerable. However in 8% treatment is instituted and quality of life assessment indicates that although pain control has been achieved overall quality of life is unchanged. In 1% there is severe disabling anaesthesia dolorosa. It will be seen that this complication is only apparent in patients without recurrence, though we have seen it 'revealed' in patients undergoing MVD with recurrent TGN after radiofrequency lesioning.

The procedure is regarded as safe, but is not completely without risk. It involves intermittent anaesthesia in an elderly patient; meningitis, and carotico-cavernous fistulae are amongst reported complications.

**4. Glycerol.** A needle is again placed into the foramen ovale and then glycerol introduced under fluoroscopic control. Accurate positioning of the needle is important. The technique has caused much controversy. In the hands of its proponents excellent results are obtained (best reports being 90% pain free at 1 year); however others report poor results (only 17% pain free at 5 years at worst) with significant dysaesthesia rates, the latter reaching 44% in some series.

**5. Balloon microcompression.** The procedure is performed under general anaesthesia. A Fogarty catheter is passed into Meckel's cavity and inflated for between 1–6 min. The method has been used since the 1950s. Sensory impairment is produced though mild. The best reported results indicate recurrence of around one third of cases, though many reports have a much lower success rate, with a dysaesthesia rate of around 10%.

## Surgical management

**1. Microvascular decompression (MVD) of the trigeminal nerve.** Microvascular decompression for trigeminal neuralgia was first carried out by Dandy in the 1930s though the operation was popularized by Jannetta more recently (1967).

**2. Fitness for surgery.** Fitness for surgery has been a major issue in the past, particularly in view of the age range with which this condition is often associated. With modern anaesthesia very few patients are unsuitable for this procedure, and the choice between percutaneous radiofrequency lesioning and MVD can be based on the outcomes of the procedures. Series of elderly patients exist in which there is little difference in outcome or morbidity comparing the over-75 age group to those younger. It is worth remembering that radiofrequency lesioning also involves anaesthesia.

**3. Operation.** This is performed via a retro-mastoid craniectomy; the subsequent approach is over the surface of the cerebellum until the nerve is identified. Arteries must be dissected free and held clear from the nerve using a small piece of Ivalon sponge or Teflon; if a vein is the cause it may be coagulated and divided. If no vessel is found a partial sensory rhizotomy gives good relief, and being a centrally placed lesion appears less likely to give rise to anaesthesia dolorosa.

**4. Risks.** In most published series the serious morbidity (death or major stroke) is significantly below 1%. The operation, being performed near to the acoustic nerve, also carries a risk of hearing impairment, possibly due to traction on the nerve whilst retracting structures to gain access to the deeper trigeminal nerve. Since brain stem auditory evoked responses have been used as a monitoring device per-operatively, the risk of unintentional hearing deficit has been reduced to about 2–3% from historical series where risks might be as high as 13%.

**5. Outcomes.** Overall, of those with clear arterial compression, a good long-term result will be obtained in about 90%, of whom some 70% are completely pain free up to 20 years post-operatively. Results of venous compression are less good as are the outcomes following partial rhizotomy – approximately 60–70% at two year follow-up. Case selection is important as poor outcomes from MVD are found in patients with atypical pain or in whom the diagnosis is not TGN. This is why the MRI findings must not be used to confirm the diagnosis – 10% of controls will show contact.

**6. Stereotactic radiosurgery.** Some controversy surrounds the results for this technique, in which focused radiation is applied to the root entry zone using the 'gamma knife'. Unfortunately the tendency of units is to report results as 'good' and not specifically stating the true 'pain-free' outcome rate used in other techniques. When this stricter criterion is used then results are less impressive; the best results find only 65% of patients experience pain relief by six months rising to 75% at 33 months. From this it will be seen that the effect is not immediate; furthermore only 56% of those who obtain relief also had complete or partial relief at five years follow-up implying a high recurrence rate. Finally it has also been demonstrated that there is a dysaesthesia rate; also a dose-related post-radiation numbness.

**7. Choice of technique.** The author considers MVD to be the treatment of choice in most instances of severe trigeminal neuralgia whilst recognizing that others may consider that it is a treatment best reserved for failed medical management or may prefer percutaneous nerve lesion technique. MVD corrects a structural abnormality and allows neurophysiological function to return to normal. In all other methods, such as radiofrequency lesion techniques, long-term nerve damage is sustained. These points summarize the reasoning:

- The natural history is for the condition to worsen.
- The side-effects of medical management, particularly cognitive, are significant and many patients fail this treatment.
- All destructive lesions (peripheral, foramen ovale, radiosurgery) are associated with a significant recurrence rate; incidence of sensory deficit and production of unpleasant dysaesthetic symptoms or even anaesthesia dolorosa.
- MVD is demonstrated to be effective and of low risk even in the elderly population.
- MR imaging can detect neurovascular compression pre-operatively so that patients with arterial compression can be advised of the likelihood of an excellent outcome, and patients can be offered an alternative technique if the scan is negative.

Although some good outcomes have been seen following radiofrequency lesioning more than one series reports that 25–50% only are pain free at 2 years in contrast to MVD where 60–70% pain free outcomes at 20 years are reported. Over a shorter time period 44% of patients were pain free at two years following balloon microcompression, while similar figures for RF lesioning were 58% and 75% for MVD. Recent evidence suggests that MVD is followed by normalization of trigeminal somatosensory physiology and cutaneous sensation; thus while trauma to the nerve can be effective (for example, partial rhizotomy), MVD itself should be regarded as a non-destructive procedure for pain relief.

## Trigeminal neuralgia as an emergency

Occasionally patients present as an emergency with pain. The patient is drowsy and ataxic having by this point taken so much carbamazepine as to suffer severe toxic effects; and is furthermore dehydrated being unable to swallow fluids owing to this action triggering the neuralgia.

Management requires admission and bed rest for the ataxia; intravenous fluids to correct dehydration and finally measures to treat the pain. An intravenous loading dose of either phenytoin or sodium valproate is usually effective in treating the pain. This may be followed by emergency MVD or if MR imaging is negative for compression one of the foramen ovale methods.

## Glossopharyngeal neuralgia

In reality the anatomy of the lower cranial nerves is such that the glossopharnygeal nerve may be considered as the upper part of a complex which includes itself, the vagus and the cranial part of the accessory nerve.

The syndrome may be considered as identical to trigeminal neuralgia except in two or three aspects. Firstly it is considerably rarer and secondly the distribution of the pain is in the area of the glossopharyngeal nerve. Thus the shooting pain is more within the throat, and triggering is also from the back of the throat. Treatment is identical; first-line drug being carbamazepine, and surgical decompression providing much the same results as for trigeminal neuralgia. There is no equivalent of radiofrequency lesioning in this condition.

## VII/VIII complex

Hemifacial spasm, tinnitus and nervus intermedius neuralgia arise from this complex. Microvascular decompression is effective for hemifacial spasm, which is the most common manifestation of compression at this level. The procedure for tinnitus is rarely performed and controversial, whilst pure nervus intermedius neuralgia is extremely rare. It can present with otalgia or throat pain. When the predominant pain is in the ear canal it has been termed geniculate neuralgia.

## Further reading

Barker FG, 2nd, Jannetta PJ, Bissonette DJ, Larkins MV, Jho HD. The long-term outcome of microvascular decompression for trigeminal neuralgia. *New England Journal of Medicine*, 1996; **334:** 1077–83.

Meaney JF, Eldridge PR, Dunn LT *et al.* Demonstration of neurovascular compression in trigeminal neuralgia with magnetic resonance imaging. *Journal of Neurosurgery*, 1995; **83:** 799–805.

Nurmikko TJ, Eldridge PR. Trigeminal neuralgia – pathophysiology, diagnosis and current treatment. *British Journal of Anaesthesia*, 2001; **87:** 117–32.

Tronnier VM, Rasche D, Hamer J *et al.* Treatment of idiopathic trigeminal neuralgia: comparison of long-term outcome after radiofrequency rhizotomy and microvascular decompression. *Neurosurgery*, 2001; **48:** 1261–68.

## Related topics of interest

Facial pain (p. 77); Headache (p. 82); Neuropathic pain – an overview (p. 113); Therapy – anticonvulsants (p. 158); Therapy – nerve blocks: somatic and lesion techniques (p. 179).

# NEUROPATHIC PAIN – AN OVERVIEW

*Andrew Severn*

## Clinical description

The traditional neuroanatomical model of the sensory system for pain fails to explain a variety of pain syndromes that are associated with damage to the sensory nerve, or the pathways through dorsal horn to cortex. Likewise, the gate control model of pain, useful as it is for explaining the modulating effect of large fibre stimulation on the pain of acute injury, fails to account for the way in which light touch may provoke pain after nerve injury. After nerve injury, it could be said that the 'gate' of the gate control model is jammed open. Similarly, therapies that work well for nociceptive pain may fail to work in neuropathic pain, or may make pain worse. There are many clinical syndromes in which pain is associated with nerve damage. Broadly similar findings are experienced with damage at any point of the nervous system, either peripheral or central, and the pain can be extremely severe, leading the clinician to resort to drastic therapies. The phenomenon of neuropathic pain is found with the following clinical syndromes:

- Surgical scar pain.
- Diabetic neuropathy.
- The complex regional pain syndromes.
- Post-herpetic neuralgia.
- Polyneuropathies and neuralgia.
- Demyelination.
- Radicular pain associated with prolapsed intervertebral disc.
- Spinal cord injury.
- Stroke.

Although there may be many mechanisms of nerve damage, and different nerves may be damaged in different conditions, there are common clinical features which are absolutely characteristic of the pathology. They may be present to varying degrees in a neuropathic pain condition.

- Spontaneous pain, which may be paroxysmal.
- Quality described as burning, shooting, numb.
- Severe pain in response to a noxious stimulus (hyperalgesia).
- Severe pain in response to a stimulus which is not normally noxious (allodynia).
- Severe pain in response to stimulation despite sensory impairment (hyperpathia).

A common complaint is of an area of skin which 'hurts though it is numb'. Other, unusual and graphic descriptions may be offered for the pain which is experienced as a familiar, but inexplicable, sensation.

## Peripheral mechanisms in neuropathic pain

Peripheral nerve damage, regardless of aetiology, results in damage to nociceptor and mechanoreceptor fibres as well as damage to the efferent motor and autonomic nerves. Axons themselves are not normally sensitive to pressure but will become so in the presence of inflammation or tissue damage. The dorsal root ganglion has its own nerve supply of nociceptors which respond to stimuli in the vicinity of the nerve root.

The damaged primary afferent fibre demonstrates three electrophysiological features:

- Spontaneous activity.
- Exaggerated response to stimulus.
- Sensitivity to catecholamines.

Spontaneous activity can develop at the site of damage, at a site of demyelination, or within the cell body of the damaged neurone in the dorsal root ganglion. Where damage to a neurone is incomplete the primary afferent terminal itself may become spontaneously active. Spontaneous activity is influenced by the local environment: inflammatory mediators and noradrenaline increase the level of activity.

As well as the ultrastructural changes that can be observed in damaged nerves, other disturbances of function are noted. These changes are associated with the production of neurokinins such as nerve growth factor. There are other biochemical changes, most notably reduction of substance P and calcitonin gene-related peptide (CGRP) synthesis, and increased neurosubstance y and vasoactive intestinal peptide synthesis. An inflammatory response occurs. Undamaged nerve fibres are themselves sensitized by changes in adjacent damaged fibres: some of the more painful neuropathies are partial nerve lesions.

## Central mechanisms in neuropathic pain

*1.  The spinal cord.*   The changes in the spinal cord neurones after nerve damage are similar to those that occur with constant low-intensity C fibre nociceptive input. The common end result of each mechanism is a state of hyperexcitability of the dorsal horn neurone. The technical term for this is central sensitization, and it has been studied in experimental models of both nociceptive and neuropathic pain. 'Windup' refers to the specific action of C fibres (that is nociceptive input) on the dorsal horn neurone. It results in a state of hyperexcitability that is so similar to that resulting from a peripheral neuropathic cause that it is helpful to consider it here. It is not known whether windup is a normal protective response or a pathological one, and therefore whether it can be classed in its own right as a cause of 'neuropathic' pain. What is clear however, is that under certain circumstances, unremitting nociceptive stimulation of the spinal cord leads to irreversible changes in the synaptic and cellular organization of the dorsal horn that persist after withdrawal of the stimulus.

*2.  The physiology of windup*   C fibres release peptides (substance P and neurokinin A) and amino acids (glutamate and aspartate) on to dorsal horn neurones. Dorsal horn neurones have receptors for neurokinin and glutamate, the latter being the $N$-methyl-D-aspartic acid (NMDA) receptor. The NMDA receptor has to be activated before it is able to interact with the glutamate transmitter. This activation is accomplished by the interaction of substance P with the neurokinin receptor. Thus the release of substance P leads to the recruitment of a second receptor type (NMDA). Subsequent C fibre stimulation leads to glutamate-mediated NMDA activation and an enhanced response to the stimulus, as measured by the increased discharge from dorsal horn neurones. The dorsal horn neurone is said to be sensitized. In its sensitized state secondary changes in other neurotransmitter receptor systems and membrane proteins occur. Interest has been expressed in the voltage-sensitive calcium channels (VSCC). In the resting state these ion channels are sensitive to morphine, whose action is to reduce the flow of calcium through the channel. However, this morphine sensitivity of the VSCC is lost in the neurone that is sensitized. Similarly, there are changes in the process of signalling between large fibre light touch neurones and the dorsal horn after sensitization. It is said that the changes in the nervous system with sensitization are analogous to those of early fetal development, in other words that sensitization involves a regression of neuronal signalling to a more 'primitive' type. Biochemical and protein synthesis changes after sensitization can be observed by measuring the appearance of products of the expression of the c-*fos* gene. This indicates synthesis of nerve growth factor and neurotransmitters within the sensitized neurone. Similar clinical entities may produce different symptoms in different patients. Different degrees of nerve damage and different responses to nerve damage may explain these differences. For example, the pain associated with the nerve damage of herpes zoster can be described as one of three variants. These variants have been described as:

- Irritable nociceptor subtype: damaged primary afferent nociceptors are responsible for the allodynia. There is an exaggerated response to capsaicin and adrenaline infiltration. There is little deficit in sensory thresholds, since sensory signalling still takes place.
- Deafferented allodynic subtype: primary afferents are more extensively damaged. C fibres develop neuromata, which discharge spontaneously. This leads to central sensitization of the dorsal horn. There is a selective loss of C fibres, so sensation to touch is preserved. However, the normal discharges of the surviving Aβ fibres cause the sensitized spinal cord to signal pain when stimulated by light touch.
- Deafferented non-allodynic subtype: the nerve damage is very extensive, the skin insensitive to all modalities and the pain is a consequence of central sensitization and neuronal reorganization.

Different degrees of nerve damage may be found in a dermatome, and the clinical findings may change with time. Patchy areas of denervation may be found.

*3.   The brain.*   Any model which tries to explain brain mechanisms in neuropathic pain must consider the diverse and detailed sensations of which a patient with a complete transection of the spinal cord lesion can complain. Such descriptions support the theory of a central pain generating area, part of a 'neuromatrix' within the brain responsible for both the sensation and its associated emotional and psychological sequelae, but triggered by nociceptive stimuli or inappropriate neuropathic stimuli. Thus a patient with a spinal cord transection may not only be aware of a phantom sensation such as bicycling, but may also suffer phantom muscle cramps and fatigue with time if the sensation persists.

An understanding of the concept, if not the details, of sensitization is important in understanding the chronic pain sufferer. The idea of pain being generated by abnormal nerve activity at spinal cord level or within the brain can be helpful to the patient and the professional who is exasperated by the failure of conventional explanations for pain. It is of note that the analgesic drug ketamine is an antagonist of the NMDA receptor, although it is not known, for reasons discussed above, whether such a drug has a role in the prophylaxis of neuropathic pain. Similarly, the concept of pre-emptive analgesia, for which there is little practical evidence, bases its reasoning on the thesis that inhibition of nociceptor input (and neuropathic input in the case of amputation pain) prior to trauma, will prevent the changes of sensitzation.

### Management of neuropathic pain

The following *drugs* are discussed in detail in other chapters, this list suggests a strategy for the management of neuropathic pains, starting with those that are more commonly used:

- Tricyclic antidepressants.
- Anticonvulsants.
- Capsaicin.
- Antiarrhythmics, for example, lignocaine, mexilitene.
- Alpha agonists, for example, tizanidine, clonidine.
- NMDA antagonists, for example, ketamine, amantidine.
- Ziconatide.
- Glial cell modulators, for example, propentofylline.

The following *techniques* are variously used for neuropathic pains. The details and indications of these techniques will be found in other chapters, but this list gives a rationale for the use of techniques, starting with the less invasive:

- Transcutaneous nerve stimulation.
- Sympathetic nervous system blocks.
- Guanethidine intravenous sympathectomy.
- Spinal cord stimulation.

## Further reading

Fields HL, Rowbotham MC. Multiple mechanisms of neuropathic pain: a clinical perspective. In: Gebhart GF, Hammond DL, Jensen TS (eds). *Proceedings of the 7th World Congress on Pain, Paris.* Seattle: IASP Press, 1994; pp. 437–54.

Melzack R. Central pain syndromes and theories of pain. In: Casey KL (ed.) *Pain and Central Nervous System Disease: The Central Pain Syndromes.* New York: Raven Press, 1991; 59–64.

Rowbotham MC, Pertersen KL, Fields HL. *Is post herpetic neuralgia more than one disorder?* IASP Newsletter Fall 1999, IASP Press, Seattle.

## Related topics of interest

# NOCICEPTIVE PAIN – AN OVERVIEW

*Andrew Severn*

## The challenge of chronic pain states

The sensory system for pain consists of a population of receptors, primary afferent neurones, neurones of the dorsal root of the spinal cord and a pathway to the midbrain, thalamus and cortex via the spinothalamic tract on the opposite side of the spinal cord. Knowledge of the anatomy of pain pathways (a result of studies of cases with damage to nerve pathways and experimental observation) is detailed, but understanding of how the behaviour of the sensory system for pain changes with nerve damage or persistent stimulation is rudimentary. In contrast to the other sensory systems, pain is not a line-labelled, modality-specific, hard-wired system, but one in which the relationship between input (stimulus) and output (response) is variable. This variability has led to the development of 'models', such as the gate control model to explain the sensory system for pain.

### Nociceptors

Receptors which respond to painful stimuli are termed nociceptors. They are simple nerve endings devoid of the elaborate organization found in the sensory systems for pressure and position sense. They respond to strong thermal and mechanical stimuli. Despite their similar ultrastructural appearance, they are not a homogeneous population, and their ability to propagate nerve impulses changes with their environment.

### Silent nociceptors

Silent nociceptors are nociceptors which are inactive in the resting state and apparently refractory to mechanical or electrical stimuli. However, in the presence of tissue damage or chemical mediators of inflammation these nociceptors become active. It is believed that although 'silent' from the perspective of nerve impulse propagation, these nociceptors are providing the sensory system with continuous data about the tissue environment. This information is signalled to the spinal cord via microtubular transport mechanisms in the axon.

### Primary afferent fibres

Primary afferent fibres are described as A or C fibres on the basis of microscopic appearance and velocity of conduction of electrical impulses. A fibres are larger, are well insulated by myelin, and conduct impulses at high velocity. C fibres are smaller, poorly insulated and conduct impulses slowly. The population of A fibres seen in a microscopic preparation of a nerve is subdivided by size into:

- Aα – motor nerves.
- Aβ – sensory nerves for light touch and vibration.
- Aγ – motor nerves.
- Aδ – sensory nerves for pain.

A and C fibres have different actions at the dorsal horn of the spinal cord.

## Visceral nociception

The innervation of visceral is notable for:

- Anatomical organization is complicated, with primary afferent nociceptive fibres entering the spinal cord via fibres which pass with efferent nerves of both the sympathetic (thoracic and lumbar spinal nerve roots) and parasympathetic (sacral nerve roots) divisions of the autonomic nervous system.
- Segmental representation of each system is wide and receptive fields for dorsal horn neurons large such that pain is not easily localized.
- A substantial proportion of fibres are silent nociceptive fibres. It is believed that these 'silent' nociceptors serve a monitoring function, and by an as yet incompletely understood mechanism (one which involves axonal transport mechanisms), 'sample' the environment near the nerve ending.

The somatic and the autonomic system are both involved in nociception of the abdomen and pelvis. The parietal peritoneum is innervated by intercostal and subcostal nerves. Somatic innervation to the perineum is the pudendal nerve (S2–S4). The sensory supply to the upper gastrointestinal tract travels with the sphlanchnic nerves to enter the spinal cord in the mid to low thoracic cord. In the female the autonomic nerves provide a source of visceral afferent sensation, and project to the spinal cord between T9 (for ovary) and L1 (for bladder and cervix). Ovarian afferents access the lower thoracic spinal roots via the lumbar sympathetic chain, whilst bladder and cervical afferents access the lumbar roots as the presacral nerves or hypogastric plexi. In both sexes there is identified a number of nerve plexi (named after the target organ) through which the sympathetic fibres pass to the spinal cord: the distribution of the sympathetic fibres to and from these plexi follows the blood supply to the organ. The pelvic splanchnic nerves (S2–S4) are parasympathetic sensory and motor to cervix, lower uterine segment, muscular stroma of prostate, distal urethra and bladder. The relative contribution of the two divisions of the autonomic nervous system to nociception in health and disease is unknown.

## Gate control

This model describes the relationship between nociceptive and tactile afferents in the dorsal horn as an electronic switch in order to explain the variability between input and output in the sensory system for pain. It was developed by Melzack and Wall in 1967 in order to explain the way in which the experience of pain could be modified by simultaneous stimulation from tactile afferents, as in rubbing a painful extremity. The model is also used to explain the influence of higher centres of control on the experience of pain. According to this model Aβ afferents and descending inhibitory pathways inhibit dorsal horn neurones from responding to Aδ and C fibre inputs. The model, like other models, is a description of a series of physiological and clinical obervations, and as such does not explain every clinical situation. For example, the persistence of pain to a chronic condition, and the experience of pain with light touch are not explained by the gate control model. To understand this it is necessary to develop a model which explains the changes observed after persistent nociceptive stimulation. One such model is neuronal sensitization.

## Neuronal sensitization

This model describes the end result of changes in the environment of nociceptor or dorsal horn spinal cord cell to tissue damage or persistent stimulation. It is described as 'peripheral' where it affects the primary afferent neurone and 'central' where it affects the dorsal horn. Sensitization is accompanied by characteristic clinical features, which are:

- Heightened sensitivity to painful stimulation – hyperalgesia.
- Pain in response to light touch – allodynia.
- Hypersensitivity of uninjured sites – secondary hyperalgesia.

Hyperalgesia results from a change in the receptive properties of the nociceptor to tissue injury. Secondary hyperalgesia is a consequence of the temporal and spatial summation of nociceptor input into the spinal cord. Allodynia results from a change in the signalling characteristics of the Aβ fibres.

*1.  Peripheral sensitization*  results from a change in the local receptor environment. There are several possible mediators of the process of sensitization, and they are present in areas of inflammation. They may act alone or in combination, and by direct action on the nerve ending or by a process of sensitizing the nociceptor to mechanical and thermal stimuli.

The mediators include:

- $H^+$ ions.
- $K^+$ ions.
- Bradykinin.
- Serotonin.
- Prostaglandins.
- Neurokinins.

A consequence of the process of sensitization is that myelinated Aβ fibres, those which form part of the gate control model, change their activity, and by a mechanism which is poorly understood, cease to function as inhibitors of dorsal horn activity.

*2.  Central sensitization*  describes the changes in the dorsal horn neurone when it is stimulated by the primary afferent neurone, either by a low-grade continuous C fibre stimulation of a nociceptive process, or following the increased activity from damaged nerves in neuropathic pain. A fibres cause transient changes at the synapse between primary afferent and spinal cord neurone. C fibres cause prolonged, progressive and ultimately irreversible changes. The increased excitability of the dorsal horn neurone that results from chronic repetitive C fibre stimulation has been studied in isolated spinal cord preparations where it is termed 'windup'. The clinical manifestation of this increased excitability, whether it has its origins in nociception or the increased and abnormal neurotransmitter activity of damaged nerves is called central sensitization.

## Management of nociceptive pain

The following drugs may be used. With the exception of paracetamol, which is an analgesic without anti-inflammatory properties, the drugs are discussed in detail in other chapters. The list of drugs includes (in the order in which a logical progression may be made in treating symptoms):

- Paracetamol. This does not inhibit prostaglandin synthesis in the peripheral tissues, but may exert some of its analgesic action by such a mechanism in the brain.
- Non-steroidal anti-inflammatory drugs.
- Weak opioids such as codeine.
- Combinations of codeine or dextropropoxyphene with paracetamol.
- Capsaicin.
- Strong opioids, such as tramadol, morphine, pethidine and fentanyl.

The following techniques may have a place in the management of chronic nociceptive pain:

- Transcutaneous nerve stimulation.
- Acupuncture.
- Local anaesthetic nerve blocks.
- Intra-articular injections of steroid.
- Sensory nerve radiofrequency lesions.
- Chemical destruction of nerve plexus.

## Related topics of interest

Cancer – opioid drugs (p. 56); Cancer – other drugs (p. 60); Neuropathic pain – an overview (p. 113); Therapy – anticonvulsants (p. 158); Therapy – anti-inflammatory drugs (p. 162); Therapy – nerve blocks: somatic and lesion techniques (p. 179).

# OSTEOARTHRITIS

*Kate Grady, Andrew Severn*

The specific changes in articular cartilage affected by osteoarthritis are evident in both weight-bearing and non-weight-bearing joints. These changes may be associated with pain and disability, but there is no correlation between pathological changes and symptoms. Osteoarthritis may lead to gross destruction of the joints, with little or much pain. On the other hand, pain may be reported in the absence of joint destruction. Pain may originate in the synovium or the joint capsule as well as from structures such as ligaments. Some pain may be referred pain. This may explain the discrepancy between pain and X-ray changes. The logic of using non-steroidal anti-inflammatory drugs (NSAIDs) was based on the precept that these changes were associated with active inflammation. This view has repeatedly been challenged, as inflammation is a variable feature. Furthermore the evidence of effectiveness has been limited. The animal model on which the original trials of NSAID mechanisms were performed does not have a human equivalent and is not pathologically similar to osteoarthritis. Despite this many early trials of NSAID were undertaken using osteoarthritis as a human model. Many trials compared different NSAID preparations, but few differences between drugs were found. Some trials compared NSAID with placebo, but few compared with paracetamol, a pure analgesic without anti-inflammatory properties. The evidence, such as it is, in favour of NSAID for osteoarthritis pain is tempered by the very real risk of gastrointestinal side-effects with prolonged use. The cyclo-oxygenase II inhibitors (COXIBs) have a similar effect as NSAIDs on pain associated with osteoarthritis, but considerably less gastrointestinal side-effects have been reported in controlled trials. Some increased safety may be conferred by the use of topical NSAID.

In contrast to the research effort for NSAID in osteoarthritis, there has been relatively little coordinated research about the efficacy of other treatments. The following is a summary of the available treatments for which reasonable evidence for efficacy has been sought:

- *Acupuncture.* This is commonly used, but studies comparing acupuncture with 'sham' acupuncture, where needles are placed randomly, have been inconclusive.
- *Capsaicin 0.025%.* This is effective for osteoarthritis of the knee.
- *Education* about arthritis and exercises for muscle strengthening around specific joints have been shown to be of value.
- *Glucosamine.* This preparation whose pharmaceutical status as food additive or drug has not yet been established is currently the subject of great interest. Controlled trials demonstrate a reduction in joint space narrowing, and there are reports that up to 20% of patients derive pain relief.
- *Joint lavage.* This may be performed with or without injection of steroids or hyaluronic acid: both these drugs are supported by randomized controlled trials.
- *Low-level laser therapy.* This has been assessed with a systematic review that has identified one controlled trial out of four which demonstrated benefit.
- *Transcutaneous electrical nerve stimulation.* This is effective in osteoarthritis of the knee, according to a systematic review.

It is thus useful to consider the pain management of osteoarthritis as management of a wider ranging 'pain syndrome'. Given that there is a nociceptive cause for the pain and with the proviso that other contributing factors to the pain syndrome have been addressed, it may on occasions be acceptable to use opioids on a chronic basis. The issues of social isolation, disability and depression need to be considered in the presentation.

## Further reading

Brosseau L, Welch V, Wells G *et al. Low level laser therapy for treating osteoarthritis.* Cochrane Library, Issue 4, 2000.

*Transcutaneous electrical nerve stimulation for knee arthritis.* Cochrane Library, Issue 4, 2000, Oxford.

Watson MC, Brookes ST, Kirwan JR, Faulkner A. The comparative of non-aspirin non-steroidal anti-inflammatory drugs for the management of osteoarthritis of the knee: a systematic review. In: Tugwell P, Brooks P, Wells G, de Bie R, Busi-Ferraz M, Gillespie W (eds). *Musculoskeletal Model of the Cochrane Database of Systematic Reviews.* The Cochrane Library. The Cochrane Collaboration Issue 1, Oxford: Update Software; 1997.

## Related topics of interest

Musculoskeletal pain syndromes (p. 95); Therapy – anti-inflammatory drugs (p. 162); Therapy – capsaicin (p. 171).

# OSTEOPOROSIS

*Kate Grady*

Bone is metabolically active. It is continually formed and resorbed. Osteoporosis occurs when resorption exceeds formation. This causes loss of bone, with a consequent susceptibility to fractures, loss of normal architecture of bones, postural deformities and soft tissue changes. All may result in pain. A clinical definition is made by standardized bone density measurements.

Osteoporosis can be idiopathic, with recognized risk factors, or secondary to other conditions such as cancer, liver impairment, coeliac disease or gastric surgery. Sex hormones have a significant effect on the skeleton. High-risk factors include early surgical menopause and early natural menopause. Other risks are steroid therapy, family history, thinness, lack of weight-bearing exercise, smoking and alcoholism.

Calcium is an important element of bone mineral. Adequate calcium intake and the calcium-regulating hormones, vitamin D and calcitonin protect against osteoporosis. Detailed management of osteoporosis is beyond the remit of this text, however the condition is described here for three reasons. Firstly, that the pain and disability associated with osteoporosis may be out of proportion to the pathological progression. Secondly, that the authors see patients with complications of osteoporosis and symptoms attributable to it which the existing disease-modifying approaches fail to address. Thirdly, some working knowledge of the available treatments and the effect they may have on pain is necessary.

## Acute vertebral crush fractures

The severity of pain is variable depending on the degree of collapse. Collapse starts as increased biconcavity of the horizontal surface of the vertebral bodies, often with loss of height. Pain at this stage is absent or mild and may be the result of micro-fractures or ligament or muscular strain. As the vertebral body collapses further and becomes visibly wedge-shaped, localized back pain may occur, with or without radicular pain depending on whether there is associated nerve compression. There can be associated pain from spasm of paraspinal muscles. Complete vertebral body crush causes severe back pain often accompanied by radicular and muscle spasm pain. Pain from crush fractures subsides within weeks. However repetitions of these fractures occur.

## Back pain

Back pain occurs in an estimated 70% of osteoporotic patients. In the absence of a radiological lesion other than the osteoporosis itself, it can be attributed to microfractures of the trabeculae or to generalized degenerative changes producing associated strain of interspinous ligaments and tenderness of paraspinal muscles. Osteoporotic changes may cause facet joint disease, sacroiliac arthritis or nerve compression with associated radiculopathy.

## Postural pains

Loss of bone architecture causes many deformities. The most troublesome is kyphosis caused by wedging or complete collapse of vertebral bodies. Sufferers develop a stiff painful neck from hyperextending in an attempt to hold up their head. As dorsal kyphosis progresses, undue effort is needed from cervical extensor muscles. Eventually the splenius capitis muscles become weak and the head can then only be lifted passively.

Neck pain frequently causes cervicogenic headache.

Inability to lift the neck causes the chin to be in constant contact with the chest wall. This causes soreness of the chin.

In order to look ahead, severely kyphotic patients flex the knees to enhance their angle of vision, thereby putting painful strain on to their knees.

Dorsal kyphosis causes the lower rib to abut the top of the pelvis painfully.

## Treatments

Pain arises as a complication of progressive osteoporosis, not from osteoporosis *per se*. Prevention of further deterioration and the treatment of the osteoporosis itself, a subject whose details are outside the remit of this text, is outlined below. Symptomatic treatment of pain may be necessary alongside treatment of the disease. A multidisciplinary approach between pain clinicians and physicians is recommended.

*1. Lifestyle factors.* Advice as to appropriate exercise, diet and exposure to sunlight should be given. Dietary supplements of calcium and vitamin D may be necessary. A synthetic precursor of vitamin D is available.

*2. Empirical treatments.* These are provided either in the primary care setting or by general physicians or dedicated osteoporosis physicians. Their prescription is beyond the scope of the pain clinic.

*3. Symptomatic treatments.*
- *Acute vertebral crush fractures.* Salmon calcitonin injections have been shown to improve pain relief. Bed rest may be necessary because of the pain associated with movement (incident pain). Analgesics such as codeine or morphine may be required. Their use should be carefully monitored, and they may be needed for short periods of time only. Transcutaneous electrical nerve stimulation (TENS), acupuncture and massage has been claimed to be of help. Epidural injections have been claimed to be of value where the fracture is not too far from the epidural injection site, and in cases of nerve root compression. Epidural steroid injections and paravertebral steroid injections are claimed to improve pain of root compression.
- *Postural pains.* Occupational therapy and physiotherapy support for activities of daily living can relieve some of the misery. Thoracolumbar supports have been claimed to reduce back pain.

## Related topics of interest

Back pain – medical management (p. 29); Musculoskeletal pain syndromes (p. 95); Osteoarthritis (p. 121); Therapy – nerve blocks: somatic and lesion techniques (p. 179).

# PELVIC AND VULVAL PAIN

*Kate Grady, Andrew Severn*

Gynaecological pain can be considered along with pain affecting the urinary tract because a number of syndromes with non-specific symptoms and overlapping features are described. Common nociceptive mechanisms are implicated. Difficulties in diagnosis of the patient presenting with pain in the lower abdomen may lead to extensive investigation of the genito-urinary system. Further confusion may be the consequence of the pain being referred from, or referred to the musculoskeletal system. Iatrogenic causes may confuse. An empirical approach to symptom control, such as the use of frequent courses of antibiotics for symptoms of pain on micturition, may lead to painful candidiasis.

Investigation may reveal pathology to account for the problem. The indication for, and the possible findings of, investigation is outside the scope of this book. Laparoscopy has made the diagnosis of painful pelvic conditions more specific. It has not, however, answered some essential questions, in the same way that magnetic resonance imaging of the spine has not helped the management of many back conditions. The unanswered questions concern the poor correlation between abnormal laparoscopic, cystoscopic, laboratory findings and the symptoms of pain. Any attempt to explain how patients with normal pelvic organs continue to experience pain has to consider that an incomplete diagnosis has been made, that the disturbance is physiological rather than pathological, or that psychological factors are playing a part. The existence of a painful 'phantom pelvis' following pelvic exenteration is evidence of the complexity of the mechanisms maintaining pain.

The environment of the uterine nociceptor is subject to change with the physiological processes of ovulation and menstruation. Afferents are sensitized by prostaglandins and leukotrienes, and become sensitive to pressure or ischaemia when the uterus contracts. Similarly, chemical irritation of the peritoneum sensitizes and stimulates afferents.

Uterine veins have been implicated in the pathophysiology of pelvic pain. The uterine venous system is unique in its ability to accommodate huge increases in its blood flow (in pregnancy), and in keeping with this, is a valveless system, in which distension may occur in the upright position. The finding of distended uterine veins at venography was said, prior to the era of laparoscopy, to be diagnostic of a specific condition of pelvic congestion.

## Chronic pelvic pain without obvious pathology

In a series of studies conducted in 1976–1979, pain was the commonest presentation and indication for laparoscopy at a gynaecological outpatient clinic. In one study, laparoscopy was normal in 65% of patients investigated for pain. Such findings have resulted in the description of a syndrome termed 'chronic pelvic pain without obvious pathology' (CPPWOP). Although the syndrome, as defined today, requires a laparoscopic exclusion of other pathology, it seems reasonable to equate it with the pelvic congestion syndrome described above. It presents as a dull ache, worsening before menses, and having a symmetrical distribution. Examination reveals tenderness over the ovarian point, a cyanotic cervix and tender adnexae.

Psychological examination reveals anxiety, feelings of being sexually unattractive, inability to sustain relationships, and stressful life events prior to symptoms. It is helpful to consider the condition as either a psychological disorder in which noxious stimulation plays a part, or a painful physiological disturbance. It is conveniently described as a disorder of the autonomic nervous system in which abnormal afferent activity (nociception) and efferent activity (altered blood flow) coexist.

*Management.* Case histories and open studies report that relief from pain can be obtained with oral contraceptives and nonsteroidal anti-inflammatory drugs which prevent the synthesis of prostaglandins, compounds involved in sensitization of the uterine nociceptor. A hypo-oestrogenic state is helpful for the control of the pain of endometriosis and is used for the control of pelvic pain without obvious pathology, using progesterone containing contraceptives such as medroxyprogesterone acetate. Physical interventions in the form of presacral nerve blockade via a percutaneous approach or via an open or laparoscopic surgical approach have been successfully reported. In this technique, sphincter control is preserved as the sacral nerve roots are unaffected. The contribution of psychological factors to the experience of pelvic pain is important to assess. General cognitive/behavioural approaches may be of value, but particular problems with issues involving sexual difficulties may need specialist attention.

A systematic review has analysed the randomized controlled trials for the above treatments and has concluded, from the five well-constructed trials, that medroxy-progesterone acetate is useful during the treatment phase, and that counselling with reassurance from ultrasound scanning improves mood and reduces pain. The reviewers comment that the antidepressant sertraline seems to be ineffective and that there is a need for further randomized trials in pelvic pain management.

## Pelvic adhesions

A diagnosis of this pathology can be made at laparoscopy, but a diagnosis cannot explain how some patients with dense adhesions (from pelvic inflammatory disease, endometriosis or previous surgery) have no pain and how some patients are incapacitated with pain despite few findings.

*Management.* Surgical division of adhesions has a variable success rate. A systematic review concluded that surgery was best reserved for the more serious cases of adhesions.

## Dysmenorrhoea

Primary dysmenorrhoea refers to painful periods not associated with pathology. Sensitization of uterine nociceptors is involved in the process. Secondary dysmenorrhoea is described in association with conditions such as endometriosis. The diagnosis of secondary dysmenorrhoea is outside the scope of this book, as is the specific management of the conditions associated with it.

*Management.* Both oral contraceptives and nonsteroidal anti-inflammatory drugs suppress prostaglandin synthesis and alter the chemical environment of the nociceptor. A hypo-oestrogenic environment is helpful for the prevention of endometriosis: hence the rationale for the use of oral progesterone contraceptives, the androgen danazol and gonadotrophin-releasing hormone analogues in the management of the secondary dysmenorrhoea of endometriosis. Irrespective of any surgery for the pathology itself, pain relief has been achieved by surgical section of the presacral plexus and the uterine nerves.

Systematic reviews have confirmed some benefit from uterine nerve ablation, and a longer-term benefit of presacral neurectomy, but only in respect of primary dysmenorrhoea, not in that of endometriosis. Danazol has been shown to be effective in four trials against placebo for the treatment of the pain of endometriosis. Fifteen trials comparing gonadotrophin hormone-releasing analogues with danazol failed to demonstrate a difference between the two classes of drugs in respect of pain relief or modification of disease.

## Haematuria/loin pain

The diagnosis is made by exclusion of organic causes to account for recurrent attacks of unilateral or bilateral loin pain associated with haematuria, but not explained by other pathology. Renal biopsy may show a number of features, such as mesangial proliferation, and immune complement C3 deposition in the arterioles, and arteriolar abnormalities may be demonstrated at renal arteriography, but these changes are non-specific and inconsistent. Psychological disturbance may complicate the presentation.

*Management.* Many approaches have been used for the pain of presumed renal or ureteric origin. Of the more invasive procedures, ureteric catheterization with instillation of a solution of capsaicin into the renal calyx and ureter has been described: this is said to result in a depletion of substance P from the nociceptors of the urothelium. The procedure may require prolonged epidural anaesthesia. Denervation of the kidney by removal of the renal capsule may afford relief, but the long-term results are disappointing. Pain returns or affects the opposite side. Autotransplantation has been reported to achieve good long-term results.

## Interstitial cystitis

A history of suprapubic pain, frequency, dysuria and urgency in the absence of infection, and cystometric findings of small bladder capacity and painful catheterization are features of this condition. Cystoscopic findings include petechial haemorrhages and occasionally ulceration. An increase in the number of mast cells in the bladder wall has been noted in sufferers of the condition. The condition occurs predominantly in middle-aged women and may be associated with irritable bowel syndrome. Many patients have had a hysterectomy prior to diagnosis, such that it has been suggested that this operation has been performed because of complaints of pelvic pain that were those of interstitial cystitis.

*Management.* Steroids and nonsteroidal anti-inflammatory drugs, antihistamines, heparin, long-term antibiotics, local anaesthetics, and tricyclic antidepressants have been reported to be of benefit in medical management of interstitial cystitis. Surgical management, with ablation of the vesicoureteric plexus has been reported to provide long-term relief. Behavioural therapy, aimed at reducing the level of distress and associated illness behaviour has been reported to be of value.

# Vulvodynia

The International Society for the Study of Vulvovaginal Disease defines vulvodynia as a sensation that is variously described as burning, irritation, rawness or discomfort.

Symptoms may be secondary to pathology such as:

- Dermatitis.
- Human papilloma virus.
- Lichen sclerosis.
- Psoriasis.
- Chronic candida.
- Vulval intraepithelial neoplasia.
- Vulval vestibulitis which affects younger women and causes local dyspareunia. The skin is erythematous and uninfected.
- Dysaesthetic vulvodynia which causes unremitting, burning pain. The histology is normal.

Patients with vulval pain should be seen by a gynaecologist with referral to dermatologists and genitourinary medicine physicians as seen appropriate by the gynaecologist so that causative pathology and otherwise treatable disease has been excluded. Some will have had surgical procedures such as vestibulectomy, skinning vulvectomy or simple vulvectomy which may have exacerbated the pain problem.

Although classification and treatment of vulval pain has not been clearly established, gynaecologists and dermatologists would tend to classify pain as 'with skin changes' or 'without skin changes'. The term dysaesthetic vulvodynia has been suggested to include all pain syndromes of unknown aetiology. There may be some merit in the simple classification of vulval pain into nociceptive and neuropathic categories. Even this apparently simple classification is however confused because words such as dysaesthetic and burning are suggestive of neuropathic pain. However vulval pain can be nociceptive without treatable cause.

For practical purposes pain can be thought of as:

- Nociceptive (due to conditions treated by gynaecologists, dermatologists or genitourinary physicians) or nociceptive with untreatable cause, i.e. vestibulitis (appropriately referred to the pain clinic).
- Neuropathic (appropriately referred to a pain clinic), i.e. 'dysaesthetic vulvodynia' (also termed vulvar dysaesthesia or essential vulvodynia) and pudendal neuralgia.

Nociceptive pain correlates with the category 'vulval pain with visible skin changes' and neuropathic pain with 'vulval pain with absent skin changes'. Neuropathic pain is identified by descriptors such as shooting, burning, stabbing, knife-like and by its signs – painful response to a normally non-painful stimulus such as stroking or garments (allodynia), a heightened response to a painful stimulus (hyperalgesia) and a sensory deficit in the area of pain – the deficit may be subclinical (hyperpathia).

Neuropathic pain can arise from diverse or 'unidentified' nerve damage or specifically from a neuralgia of the pudendal nerve. Allodynia, hyperalgesia and hyperpathia can be demonstrated in areas innervated by the pudendal nerve. Obvious cause e.g. trauma or infection may not be identified.

A multi-dimensional approach to pain management is recommended. The sufferer must understand that the pain is not psychological in origin. However, all pain can be affected by psychological and social factors, and vulval pain is likely to be affected by psychosexual influences. Vulval pain is thought to bear a relationship to sexual or life stress such as loss of partner, but no relationship to sexual abuse. A full psychosocial assessment with particular attention to the psychosexual is warranted.

Acupuncture and transcutaneous nerve stimulation may have a role in the treatment of vestibulitis. NSAIDs/COXIBs and/or simple analgesics may be used. Local anaesthetic creams can be prescribed to cover intercourse.

***Neuropathic vulval pain*** can be treated by antineuropathic medication such as tricyclic antidepressants – nortriptyline 10–25 mg at night or amitriptyline at same dose if agitation or sleep disturbance (average dose for improvement has been reported at 40 mg at night), anticonvulsants – gabapentin 300 mg per day increased weekly by 300 mg up to 1200 mg per day has been shown to be effective.

Some workers feel some neuropathic pains are sympathetically maintained. These may be amenable to local anaesthetic block of sympathetic chain (ganglion impar block), where pain relief effect will outlast pharmacological duration of local anaesthetic.

## Further reading

Jones RW. Vulval pain. *Pain Reviews*, 2000; **7**(1).

## Systematic reviews

Prentice A, Deary AJ, Goldbeck-Wood S, Farquhar C, Smith SK. Gonadotrophin-releasing hormone analogues for pain associated with endometriosis. *The Cochrane Library*, Issue 4, 2000, Oxford.

Selak V, Farquhar C, Prentice A, Singla A. *Danazol for pelvic pain associated with endometriosis*. The Cochrane Library, Issue 4, 2000, Oxford.

Wilson ML, Farquhar CM, Sinclair OJ, Johnson NP. Surgical interruption of pelvic nerve pathways for primary and secondary dysmenorrhoea. *The Cochrane Library*, Issue 4, 2000.

## Related topics of interest

Musculoskeletal pain syndromes (p. 95); Nociceptive pain – an overview (p. 117); Therapy – nerve blocks: autonomic (p. 176).

# POST-AMPUTATION PAIN

*Kate Grady*

Pain following limb amputation can be of many causes and is said to be an amalgam of post-operative pain, stump pain of nociceptive or neuropathic cause, phantom pain, and other pains related to disability. Careful consideration should be given to cause so treatment can be properly directed. An amputee is said to be 'established' one year following amputation and it is often not until this stage that pain clinic referral is contemplated. However there is an incidence of phantom pain of 72% as early as 8 days after surgery; therein may lie a need for the early input of the pain clinician. A total of 90% of amputees have non-painful phantom sensation 6 months after surgery. Phantom sensation and pain are a complex physiological phenomenon resulting from remapping of the sensory homunculus, occurring quickly after the physiological insult.

Although the correlation between preoperative pain and the likelihood of developing phantom pain is recognized, this is not consistent. This correlation and dramatic anecdotal evidence for the pain memory whereby phantom pain resembles the pre-op pain in location and character, has prompted studies whereby pre-op pain has been controlled by epidural injection and the effect of that on outcome has been assessed. There have been five studies which have had varying clinical protocols. No consistent evidence has been drawn for the technique.

After amputation, biomechanics are distorted and never return to normal even with the best of prosthetics. This can result in back pain, proximal arthritis (3–6 fold increase), arthritis of joints in the contralateral limb and fall-related pain.

In upper limb amputees, symptoms of overuse of the contralateral limb occur such as shoulder pain, epicondylitis and repetitive strain injury.

Pains specific to the condition are phantom pain and neuropathic pain of the stump. Causes of nociceptive pain of the stump should be sought and treated.

All pain resulting from amputation requires a full biopsychosocial assessment involving physician, physiotherapist and psychologist but also prosthetist and occupational therapist with regard to work ergonomics. Cognitions and behavioural problems may need to be addressed.

## Nociceptive pain of the stump

Nociceptive stump pain gets better over time. Fifty seven per cent have stump pain at 8 days, 22% stump pain at 6 months, the result of tissue healing.

The UK's 75 000 amputees are followed up in 27 Subregional Disablement Service Centres. Nociceptive causes of stump pain are attended to in such clinics and can be described under the following categories:

- Abnormal stump in which the myoplasty, that part of the muscle that is fashioned over the bony stump, alters its architecture and allows prominence of the stump bone.
- Adherent scars.
- Folliculitis and infected epidermoid cysts.
- Allergic contact dermatitis due to prosthetic materials or creams.
- Badly fitting prostheses.
- Sweat maceration.
- Vascular insufficiency.

Treatment of these is best carried out by a rehabilitation specialist often in conjunction with other specialists, for example, a vascular surgeon or a dermatologist.

### Neuropathic pain of the stump

Neuropathic pain of the stump may be due to neuromata or of less-specific cause. The suspicion of a neuroma can be confirmed by MR scan. Neuromata in pressure-sensitive areas can be embedded deep in tissue. This procedure is performed by plastic surgeons. The presence of a neuroma makes phantom pain more likely. Most neuropathic pain of the stump is less specific but can present floridly, symptoms of allodynia and hyperalgesia causing major difficulties with prosthetic rehabilitation.

### Phantom limb pain

Phantom pain should be clearly differentiated from phantom sensation. Sensations encompass numbness, heat, cold, itch and awareness of position, length and volume. The phantom limb tends to shorten (telescope) over time. 'Movement' can occur in the amputated portion either 'willed' or involuntary, and is associated with jumping in the stump known as stump jactitation. Phantom pain affects 75% of patients within 3 days, and persists to 2 years in 59%. It may develop years after the amputation. It is described as stabbing, shooting, squeezing, cramping and may be affected by position of the stump.

All of these phenomena can cause distress. Simple reassurance may suffice in allaying distress.

The mechanisms of phantom pain are thought to be:

- Peripheral afferent fibre sensitization and increased sensitivity to adrenaline and noradrenaline;
- An increase in general excitability at spinal cord level with normal A delta and C fibre input gaining access to a secondary group of pain signalling neurones and degeneration of C fibres. The normal spinal cord terminations of the C fibres degenerate and are then occupied by A beta fibres, which in turn signal pain sensations;
- Somatosensory remapping.

Pain is often worse with micturition, bowel evacuation and sexual intercourse suggesting an autonomic component.

Poor blood supply to and muscle tension of the stump can aggravate phantom pain. Stump jactitation may exacerbate phantom pain.

## Treatment

### Neuropathic pain of the stump

Non-pharmacological treatments include stump massage, transcutaneous electrical nerve stimulation and hypnotherapy and relaxation. Pharmacological treatments include tricyclic antidepressants, gabapentin (or those in combination), with capsaicin, lamotrigine, clonazepam, mexiletine and ketamine reserved for treatment failure. Problems are encountered with capsaicin as sweating and overheating from tight-fitting stump sock and liners cause a more intense rubifacient effect.

Lignocaine patches, when available, may have a role. Local anaesthetic injections to tender spots and neuromata have been used.

## Phantom limb pain

Non-pharmacological methods include:

- Transcutaneous electrical nerve stimulation.
- Contralateral limb exercises – if the amputated portion feels as if it is awkwardly positioned move the contralateral limb as if to relieve that awkward posture – if the amputated portion is cramping rub the contralateral limb.
- Mirror exercises – a mirror is used to visualize the image of the contralateral limb making movements as if to relieve pain, in the would-be position of the absent limb.

Pharmacological treatments, on the basis that they work in other neuropathic pains, include tricyclic antidepressants, gabapentin (or those two in combination) and, as reserve treatments, carbamezepine, lamotrigine, clonazepam and mexiletine. Ketamine has given relief as a long-term subcutaneous infusion (0.125–0.25 mg kg$^{-1}$h$^{-1}$). The author has had considerable success in the use of gabapentin. No additional benefit is conferred above 900 mg daily. Intravenous salmon calcitonin has been shown to be effective.

Tizanidine, an alpha-adrenergic agonist with a useful action in some neuropathic pains can be used to treat stump jactitation.

Spinal cord stimulation is used but there must be careful patient selection.

It may be that neuropathic pain of the stump and phantom limb pain are sympathetically maintained. Injection of local anaesthetic to sympathetic plexi may be therapeutic (stellate for arm, lumbar sympathetic chain for leg), particularly if the pain is exacerbated by poor vascularity.

## Further reading

Jensen T, Krebs B, Nielson J, Rasmussen P. Immediate and long-term phantom pain in amputees: incidence, clinical characteristics and relationship to pre-amputation pain. *Pain*, 1985; **21**: 267–78.

Nikolajsen L, Jensen TS. Phantom limb pain. *British Journal of Anaesthesia*, 2001; **87**(1).

Sherman RA, Arena JG. Phantom limb pain: mechanisms, incidence and treatment. *Critical Reviews in Physical and Rehabilitation Medicine*, 1992; **4**(1, 2): 1–26.

## Related topics of interest

Neuropathic pain – an overview (p. 113); Scars, neuromata, post-surgical pain (p. 142); Therapy – antiarrhythmics (p. 156); Therapy – anticonvulsants (p. 158); Therapy – antidepressants (p. 160); Therapy – capsaicin (p. 171); Therapy – ketamine and other NMDA antagonists (p. 173); Therapy – spinal-cord and brain stimulation (p. 198).

# POST-HERPETIC NEURALGIA

*Kate Grady*

Post-herpetic neuralgia (PHN) is a chronic pain which can occur following acute herpes zoster infection (shingles). Herpes zoster infection results from reactivation of the varicella zoster virus, dormant in perineural tissues following a primary chickenpox infection. Acute herpes zoster infection may be painful, although 40% of patients do not report pain. PHN is pain persisting after the pain of the acute infection. The demarcation between pain due to acute infection and the pain of PHN is not defined. Some define pain persisting beyond the crusting of acute infective lesions as PHN; others, pain after specified periods from 4 weeks to 6 months since the eruption of acute infective skin lesions. There is therefore no clear definition of PHN.

## Pathophysiology

Acute inflammation and ischaemia during the acute infection cause a necrotizing reaction in the dorsal root, the dorsal root ganglion and the dorsal horn. Large myelinated fibres are more extensively damaged and are reduced in number. This allows increased transmission of nociceptive information at the dorsal horn and thereby pain. The elderly have fewer large myelinated fibres. Further reduction in number by disease process explains the susceptibility of the elderly to the development of PHN. Usually only a single dermatomal segment is affected. Damage occurs to both sensory and motor nerves but the effect on motor nerves is subclinical.

## Clinical features

If PHN is defined as pain persisting at 1 month, the incidence varies from 9% to 14%. It has been found to be only 3% at 1 year and tends to gradually improve and eventually remit. More severe pain lasts longer. PHN develops almost exclusively in people over the age of 50. It occurs in up to 65% of those over the age of 60. Acute herpes zoster causes pain in a dermatomal distribution. The pain of PHN is in the dermatomal distribution of the acute infection. The commonest sites for PHN are thoracic dermatomes and the ophthalmic division of the trigeminal nerve. It is less common with lumbar dermatomal involvement. It is usually unilateral.

Pain is a constant aching, burning or itching. There are paroxysms of severe stabbing or lancinating pain. Allodynia, hyperalgesia and hyperaesthesia often occur. There is scarring and pigmentation in the affected dermatomal distribution with a wider area of sensory change.

It is now clear that the various manifestations of PHN are the consequence of varying degrees of sensory nerve damage. Thus three 'subtypes' have been described, and distinguished both by clinical features and the response to treatment:

- irritable nociceptor subtype: damaged primary afferent nociceptors are responsible for the allodynia. There is an exaggerated response to capsaicin and adrenaline infiltration. There is little deficit in sensory thresholds, since sensory signalling still takes place.

- deafferented allodynic subtype: primary afferents are more extensively damaged. C fibres develop neuromata, which discharge spontaneously. This leads to central sensitization of the dorsal horn. There is a selective loss of C fibres, so sensation to touch is preserved. However, the normal discharges of the surviving Aβ fibres cause the sensitized spinal cord to signal pain when stimulated by light touch.
- deafferented non-allodynic subtype: the nerve damage is very extensive, the skin is insensitive to all modalities and the pain is a consequence of central sensitization and neuronal reorganization.

Pain can be severe enough to cause lethargy, anorexia, sleep disturbance, loss of libido and consideration of suicide.

## Management

*Prevention.* Currently there is no proven useful therapy for the prevention of PHN. The benefits of acyclovir and corticosteroids require further evaluation. Therefore vigorous efforts must be made to prevent acute herpes zoster infection by vaccination programmes, etc. Opinion is divided as to the role of nerve blocks. Amitriptyline has been suggested as a prophylactic drug.

## Treatment

*1.* *Tricyclic antidepressants.* Systematic review of tricyclic antidepressants has concluded a benefit for the treatment of PHN, with a NNT quoted as 2.3 for 50% pain relief at 3–6 weeks. Several drugs of the same category may need to be tried. Amitriptyline is recommended at an initial dose of 10 mg nocte in the over-65 age group and at 25 mg nocte for those under 65.

*2.* *Capsaicin.* The combined NNT from two trials of capsaicin 0.075% has been calculated to be 5.3. The use of capsaicin, however, is inappropriate in the presence of 'irritable nociceptor' PHN.

*3.* *Anticonvulsants.* Gabapentin has been shown to reduce the pain of PHN. Reports of efficacy of carbamazepine and phenytoin have also been made.

*4.* *Opioids.* There is some evidence to support partial effectiveness of opioid drugs in PHN. Morphine has been shown to significantly relieve PHN and results are favourable for another strong opioid agonist, oxycodone.

*5.* *Local anaesthetic.* Daily subcutaneous injections of local anaesthetic have been reported. This technique may be particularly appropriate for the 'irritable nociceptor' subtype of PHN. Repeated somatic nerve blocks and sympathetic blocks have also been reported. The rationale is the alteration of central sensitivity by the reduction of nociceptive and peripheral neuropathic input into the dorsal horn.

*6.* *Steroids.* Steroids are claimed to be effective both in painful peripheral lesions, and around the nerve root, where reduction of inflammatory processes may prevent neuronal damage.

**7.  *Transcutaneous nerve stimulation.*** The benefit of TENS is dependent on there being sufficient innervation from normally conducting fast fibres. In practice, TENS is poorly tolerated where there is extensive allodynia.

## Further reading

Rowbotham M, Harden N, Stacey B. Gabapentin for the treatment of postherpetic neuralgia: a randomized controlled trial. *JAMA*, 1998; **280:** 1837–42.

Rowbotham MC, Pertersen KL, Fields HL. Is post herpetic neuralgia more than one disorder? *IASP Newsletter*, Fall, 1999; IASP Press, Seattle.

## Systematic reviews

Lancaster T, Silagy C, Gray S. Primary care management of acute herpes zoster: systematic review of evidence from randomized controlled trials. *British Journal of General Practice*, 1995; **45:** 39–45.

McQuay HJ, Tramer M, Nye BA, Carroll D, Wiffen PJ, Moore RA. A systematic review of antidepressants in neuropathic pain. *Pain*, 1996; **68:** 217–27.

Schmader KE, Studenski S. Are current therapies useful for the prevention of postherpetic neuralgia? A critical analysis of the literature. *Journal of General Internal Medicine*, 1989; **4**(2): 83–9.

Volmink J, Lancaster T, Gray S, Silagy C. Treatments for postherpetic neuralgia: a systematic review of randomized control trials. *Family Practice*, 1996; **13**(1): 84–91.

Zhang WY, Li Wan Po A. The effectiveness of topically applied capsaicin: a meta-analysis. *European Journal of Clinical Pharmacology*, **46:** 517–22.

## Related topics of interest

Neuropathic pain – an overview (p. 113); Nociceptive pain – an overview (p. 117); Therapy – antidepressants (p. 160); Therapy – capsaicin (p. 171); Therapy – spinal-cord and brain stimulation (p. 198); Therapy – TENS, acupuncture and laser stimulation (p. 206).

# PREGNANCY

*Kate Grady*

Pain in pregnancy is very common and it is important to reassure when appropriate but still recognize potentially serious conditions such as a developing placental abruption in a patient who has complained of non-specific abdominal pain all through pregnancy. A common reason to be rushed into delivering early is undiagnosed abdominal pain sometimes associated with heart-burn or vomiting.

Pain in pregnancy takes away from what should be an enjoyable experience and pain which goes untreated can result in premature delivery, either spontaneous or induced. The management of pain in pregnancy has to balanced with fetal well-being. Pains are precipitated either directly or indirectly by pregnancy.

These are due to the mechanical and hormonal effects of pregnancy, due to the modification of other disease by the pregnancy, and due to delivery and procedures undertaken for delivery. Pains of pre-existing conditions may become more symptomatic during pregnancy because treatment has had to be restricted for fetal reasons. A fresh treatment strategy may need to be employed. Because options for treatment are not as plentiful as in the non-pregnant state and because some of these pains are peculiar to the pregnant state, each is given special consideration so therapeutic potential can be maximized. Before deciding on therapies what is available in terms of fetal safety must be defined.

## Treatment

The non-pharmacological methods have an advantage over pharmacological because of fetal safety. If drugs are to be used non-pharmacological methods may provide dose-reducing adjuncts. Drugs may cover a period in which a non-pharmacological method is getting to work. The first trimester is the time of greatest risk to the developing fetus.

*1. Non-pharmacological methods.* Physiotherapy can address muscle tension problems, pain problems resulting from altered biomechanics, can facilitate mobilization and can provide sacroiliac belts for the treatment of symphisis pubis diastasis pain, although these are not tremendously helpful.

TENS is used to treat back pain, pains precipitated by muscle tension, headaches and nerve entrapment. The abdominal wall is avoided as a site for placement of pads to avoid uterine stimulation and the theoretical potential for inducing labour.

Acupuncture is used for the treatment of headache, nerve entrapment pain and back pain. There is a theoretical risk of uterine stimulation but there are no reports of this in the literature.

Water gymnastics (aqua-aerobics) during the second half of pregnancy have been shown to significantly reduce the intensity of back pain.

Stressful social and psychological factors should be addressed.

*2. Pharmacological methods.* Drugs must be carefully selected and attention given to the timing of the fetus's exposure to the drug. The dose and duration of exposure should be minimized. Because of the ethics of research in pregnancy there are no controlled studies in pregnant women. The drugs which are used are ones in which animal studies have failed to demonstrate a fetal risk or have shown an adverse effect that was not confirmed in controlled studies in women in the first trimester.

Drugs for which there is positive evidence of human fetal risk and likelihood of causing fetal abnormalities outweighs any benefit should be avoided.

### 1. Nociceptive pain treatments.

- *Paracetamol.* There are no reports of congenital abnormalities attributed to para-cetamol. Fetal death has been reported in maternal overdose.
- *Aspirin and non-steroidal anti-inflammatory drugs (NSAIDs).* The use of these drugs in the third trimester is associated with premature closure of the ductus arteriosus. There is a risk of neonatal haemorrhage which is of particular concern in the neonate. Low-dose NSAIDs in the second trimester are associated with oligohydramnios. The above risks do not appear to apply to low-dose aspirin as used in pre-eclampsia.
- *Opioids.* Use of codeine in the first trimester is associated with respiratory malformations, congenital heat disease and cleft lip and palate. In the first and second trimesters it is associated with inguinal and umbilical hernias and a neonatal withdrawal syndrome is described.

Dextropropoxyphene is associated with a neonatal withdrawal syndrome.

Morphine is safely used for short-term interventions. Most of the available long-term data are for methadone which is associated with good maternal and fetal outcome and has the advantage of being an NMDA antagonist and therefore having some antineuropathic activity. Long-term users must continue their regular daily dose whilst in labour. Epidural analgesia may be used for the superimposed pain of labour (including epidural opioids) as tolerance to opioids will be a problem. There will be an increase in analgesic requirements after operative delivery which can be provided for by epidural or intravenous opioid infusion. Dose equivalents between drugs and routes of administration are unpredictable so the effect of any super-imposed analgesic intervention needs to be very carefully monitored.

- *Triamcinolone* (10mg) in an equal mix of 1% lignocaine and 0.5% bupivacaine up to 20 ml has been used to treat coccydynia, neuromata and nerve entrapment pain.

### 2. Neuropathic treatments.

- *Amitriptyline.* Limb reduction abnormalities have been reported from using amitriptyline in the first trimester. In 500 000 second and third trimester pregnancies there were no reports of fetal abnormalities.
- *Anticonvulsants.* There are no data available for gabapentin but all other anticonvulsants commonly used in pain management are thought to be unsafe.

## Breast feeding

Paracetamol and diclofenac enter breast milk but in such small doses they are thought to be clinically insignificant. Morphine enters breast milk but neonatal effect is limited because of low bioavailability. Amitriptyline enters breast milk and there are reports of neonatal drowsiness which ceases on stopping the amitriptyline.

### Management

Multidisciplinary pain management is of importance and medical input should include obstetric and neonatology opinions where necessary. There should be a close link to a psychiatrist as depression is linked to pain and depression is a risk in the postnatal period.

Patients may require management into the postnatal period if their pain persists or even if it has abated for advice as to weaning off their medication and management of potential future problems.

# Pains

The management of pain in pregnancy requires the joint input of obstetrician and pain clinician not least so complications of pregnancy can be differentiated from pain syndromes. Reluctance to carry out X-ray investigations should not cause oversight of pain problems of sinister cause such as those due to developing malignancy. Several of the following pains can co-exist but each requires separate consideration.

### Back pain

An element of back pain is normal during pregnancy. Half of all pregnant patients report back pain at some stage. It results from the lordosis that develops because of the enlarged anterior mass of the uterus. It may also be contributed to by increased laxity in sacroiliac, sacrococcygeal and symphysis pubis joint induced by relaxin. Serious sinister and systemic causes must be excluded. Pre-existing back pain often worsens in severity and frequency of symptoms. Asymptomatic disc herniation is common in pregnancy. 1:10000 pregnant women will develop radicular symptoms. Pregnancy appears to be a risk factor for postpartum disc prolapse. Spondylolisthesis may be caused by increased joint laxity.

*Treatments.* Advice on movement, mobility and lifting should be offered. A systematic review has shown that specially shaped pillows appear to reduce back pain and promote sleep in late pregnancy. Education, support and advice and non-pharmacological methods such as a trochanteric belt and manipulation for sacro-iliac pain are used. Paracetamol and opioids can be employed. If radicular pain occurs beyond the first trimester amitriptyline or epidural triamcinolone may help.

### Coccydynia

Coccydynia is associated with alteration in ligament laxity and changes in posture which occur during pregnancy. It is exacerbated by sitting and may be worse in the post-partum period after prolonged sitting during labour. Delivery may cause trauma to the coccyx. There are reports of pre-existing coccydynia being exacerbated by pregnancy. There may be a case in these patients for elective Caesarean section as potential trauma of delivery may exacerbate pain further.

*Treatments.* Non-pharmacological methods, paracetamol, opioids, injection of steroid to caudal epidural space, coccygeal joints and ganglion impar can be used alone or in combination.

### Post-partum back pain

Back pain of pregnancy continues after delivery for longer than 6 months in an estimated 43%. It is worse in the younger multigravid patient with a pre-pregnancy history of back pain.

The relationship of back pain to epidurals is debated. The postulation that loss of normal posture and sensation to posture may contribute to the development or exacerbation of back pain has been discounted on the basis that pain is not related to the degree of motor block. The site of epidural puncture can be exquisitely tender in that very localized area. Some have a more widespread area of ache or bruised-like feeling surrounding the point of insertion. Epidural abscess must be excluded.

*Treatments* for generalized back pain as above; for localized back pain at puncture site, topical nonsteroidal anti-inflammatory preparations, low-level laser therapy.

Physiotherapy should be instituted surrounding the time of epidural blood patching as there are reports of increased backache after the procedure, likely related to immobility.

### Symphysis pubis diastasis pain

Relaxation of the pelvic ligaments occurs to allow for more movement of the symphysis pubis. This can occur to the point of widening of the symphysis pubis and instability of the pelvis. There is no evidence however that the degree of symphyseal distraction is related to the amount of pelvic pain. Weight bearing at the symphysis pubis produces movement which is painful, with associated muscle spasm and neuropathic pain caused by tension and pressure on the nerves in the region; sciatica and genitofemoral neuralgia (pain in groin and labia) are associated. The pain often resolves in the few weeks after delivery.

*Treatment.* TENS, physiotherapy, sacroiliac belts, paracetamol, amitriptyline and opioids are used. There is a patient support group.

### Recurrent loin pain and dysuria without positive microbiology culture

Intermittent loin pain starting in the second or third trimester has been attributed to the enlarging uterus compressing the ureters as they cross the pelvic brim (right side more common than the left). Ureteric dilatation has been demonstrated in the absence of renal stones and the patient gets relief from being on her hands and knees.

*Treatment.* Heat packs and TENS may be of use. Morphine is used for exacerbations and amitriptyline and diclofenac have been used for prophylaxis. Diclofenac should be avoided after 34 weeks or if there is any renal compromise.

### Upper abdominal pain

Enlargement of the abdomen causes stretching of the abdominal wall which causes both muscular pain and tension on nerves which travel within causing pain. The anterior branches of the anterior rami of the thoracic nerves pierce rectus abdominis. Stretching of rectus abdominis can cause unilateral pain in the distribution of a thoracic nerve extending to the midline. At the point of its emergence from the costal margin the nerve is exquisitely tender. Pain and tenderness are quite common over the edges of the lower ribs where the abdominal muscles insert. Upper abdominal discomfort can also arise from the rounded head of a breech pressing against the ribs. These must be clearly differentiated from upper abdominal pain of pre-eclampsia.

*Treatment.* Non-pharmacological methods and injection of local anaesthetic and steroid at the point of its emergence from the costal margin may be effective.

## Pelvic and lower abdominal pain

Similarly stretching of the lower abdominal wall can cause pain in the distribution of the iliohypogastric nerve causing pain above the inguinal ligament, ilioinguinal nerve, causing pain in the medial thigh, genitofemoral nerve causing pain in the groin and/or labia, and the lateral cutaneous nerve of thigh causing pain in the lateral thigh (meralgia paraethetica). Pain is quite often felt in the anterior upper thigh.

*Treatment.* Non-pharmacological methods and injection to tender points. A neuropathic pain in an area from above pubic bone to above umbilicus has been described. It is thought that this may be a pain maintained by sympathetic supply to the uterus.

## Carpal tunnel syndrome

Hand symptoms due to compression of either median or ulnar nerves occur. They are more common in pregnancy because of fluid retention, fat deposition and relaxation of the transverse carpal ligaments by relaxin.

*Treatment.* Removal of constricting devices, elevation of the limb and the use of splints may help. Surgical release is a last resort.

## Headaches

Recurrent headaches tend to improve during pregnancy. They may not however, and patients may be rendered worse because treatment is contraindicated e.g. sumatriptan is withdrawn because it is known to cause fetal malformations in rabbits. Systemic diseases should be excluded as causes.

*Treatment.* Non-pharmacological methods should be used if possible. Paracetamol is the mainstay of treatment.

## Postdural puncture headache

*Treatment.* Conservative treatment comprises high oral fluid intake and simple analgesics. Persistent headaches are often treated with an epidural blood patch with a success rate of 85–90%. This invasive procedure is not free from complications and is contraindicated in patients with meningitis, systemic infection, coagulopathy, cutaneous lumbar lesions and those receiving anticoagulant therapy. Numerous drug therapies have been reported in the literature as alternatives including sumatriptan a 5-HT1δ agonist at a dose of 6 mg subcutaneously and repeated 2 h later and again 9 h later to obtain complete relief.

### Neuropraxia

This can be caused by direct needle trauma at the time of regional block or by insertion of the epidural catheter. It can also be caused by birth trauma associated with prolonged labour and cephalopelvic disproportion. It can occur from undue pressure on nerves such as lithotomy position causing trauma to common peroneal nerve, prolonged hip flexion and abdominal oedema causing trauma to the lateral cutaneous nerve of thigh. It is important to exclude an epidural abscess as the cause. Careful examination, early involvement of neurologists and early recourse to MR scanning is important.

### Perineal pain and dyspareunia

These can be caused by neuromata or painful swollen scars.

*Treatment.* A systematic review has reported that further evidence is required to evaluate the use of ultrasound although some trials reported improvement in pain. Other treatments comprise non-pharmacological, infiltration to scar of local anaesthetic and steroid, amitriptyline, surgical revision if appropriate.

### Pain in Caesarean section scar

This may be due to trapping of nerve within layers of scar or due to the development of neuromata. Treatments can be applied as for perineal scars.

Other pains include intractable heart-burn and pain from damage associated with a transient osteoporosis of pregnancy. Back pain and hip pain are common, fractures have been reported during delivery and patients may lose height. It is unclear whether reduction in bone density bears any relationship to pelvic and back pain occurring in pregnancy.

### Change in disease due to pregnant state

Rheumatoid arthritis tends to go into remission during pregnancy so the need to prescribe NSAIDs may vanish. Disease-modifying antirheumatic drugs (DMARDs) such as methotrexate and sulfasalazine may be withheld if remission occurs.

Ankylosing spondylitis usually does not change during pregnancy.

## Further reading

Roche S, Hughes EW. Pain problems associated with pregnancy and their management. *Pain Reviews*, 1999; **6**.

## Systematic reviews

Hay-Smith EJC. *Therapeutic ultrasound for postpartum perineal pain and dyspareunia (Cochrane review).* In: The Cochrane Library, Issue 4, 2000. Oxford: Update software.

Young G, Jewell D. *Interventions for preventing and treating backache in pregnancy (Cochrane Review).* In: The Cochrane Library, Issue 4, 2000. Oxford: Update software.

# SCARS, NEUROMATA, POST-SURGICAL PAIN

*Kate Grady*

Chronic pain after surgery is an important and underestimated cause of morbidity. There are several potential causes, and they are discussed here. Nociceptive and neuropathic mechanisms may be involved. An understanding of the nature of chronic pain and the likely cause is important to managing the condition – for example, fear of recurrent disease may be an important factor in the presentation.

## Scar pain

Hypertrophic scars regress with time. Gross keloid scars may be suitable for excision. Excision is however almost always followed by a recurrence. Steroid creams and pressure on scars have been used to prevent recurrence. Steroid injections may be more effective. Revision of painful scars is not always successful in producing pain relief and should be undertaken with reservation. It is suggested, but not proven, that prevention of secondary CNS changes by local anaesthetic block can result in less pain after surgery.

Infiltration of the scar with local anaesthetic and steroid (e.g. bupivacaine 0.25–0.5% with depomedrone 20–40 mg with attention to local anaesthetic toxic doses) has been reported as effective. Cryotherapy to the scar is effective in isolated scar pain. Benefit from sympathetic nerve blocks suggests that pain may have a sympathetic component. Subsequent treatments are repeated sympathetic nerve blockade and the use of drugs which act on the sympathetic nervous system.

Tricyclic antidepressant drugs, anticonvulsants and membrane-stabilizing agents are all used. Radiofrequency lesioning locally to the scar or to the dorsal root ganglion is another option. Such lesions may be more appropriately made with low-temperature (pulsed) radio-frequency techniques.

## Neuromata

Neuropathic pain is pain caused by a primary lesion or dysfunction within the nervous system. The neuroma is the animal model for neuropathic pain. In humans neuromata can cause pain. Neuromata develop following partial transection of a nerve. The initial pain is from A$\delta$ and C fibres firing. An increase in neuronal excitability causing spontaneous discharge of action potential can occur following nerve transection. Ongoing pain, accompanied by allodynia, hyperalgesia and hyperpathia then occurs.

### Pathophysiology

- When a nerve axon is cut the part which is still attached to the cell body forms a swelling (end bulb). Elongating processes are sprouted from the end bulb as an attempt to regenerate. Regeneration occurs if the axonal sprouts reach their target peripheral receptors and normal function is restored. If the processes do not reach their target sprouting continues and when their forward progress is blocked sprouts become entangled to form a neuroma. Sprouts cause disruption of the myelin sheath. Secondary reorganization of membrane electrical properties takes place, causing neuronal hyperexcitability. This may be due to an increase in number of sodium channels in the proximal axonal membrane.

- Disruption of the myelin sheath produces ectopic foci of electrical activity locally and in sites remote from the damage such as the dorsal root ganglion.
- In undamaged nerves individual afferent fibres conduct independently, insulated by myelin. Where demyelination has occurred, nerves cross-excite each other electrically. This is termed as ephaptic transmission or neuronal cross-talk. When nociceptive afferents cross-excite each other, amplification of pain occurs. However, coupled fibres can be of different types; nociceptor afferents may be activated by afferents for light touch such that allodynia occurs. Ephaptic transmission occurs between afferents and efferents.
- Neuromata are chemically sensitive, for example, to adrenaline and noradrenaline.
- Neuromata discharge abnormally into the central nervous system (CNS) from the periphery. This may cause a phenomenon of central sensitization.

## Clinical features

Neuromata are present in sites where the perineurium has been breached but not at all sites where nerves have been cut. Pain from neuromata is variable and may be governed, amongst other things, by genetic factors. Neuromata are often, but not necessarily, palpable as discrete tender lumps. Several neuromata can be found, trapped at a suture line because the regenerating nerve fibres are unable to sprout across it.

- Pain is most intense during the first 2 weeks of its development, continuing beyond then but less sustained.
- Pain from neuroma may be spontaneous or provoked. Pressure on the neuroma may provoke pain through contiguous areas.
- Pain is augmented by percussion of the neuroma. The neuromata may demonstrate allodynia, hyperalgesia or hyperpathia.
- Temperature, metabolic and chemical factors can excite ectopic discharge in animal models.

## Treatments

- Systemic administration of drugs acting on the sodium channel can prevent electrical firing. First-line treatment is with anticonvulsants. Local anaesthetics and antiarrythmics are also used.
- Calcium channel blockers may also have a role in reducing excitability but have not yet been clinically evaluated.
- Surgical excision of neuromata can be effective but in susceptible individuals neuromata recur.
- Mechanically sensitive neuromata can be surgically embedded in deep tissue and in bone marrow away from factors which may encourage nerve growth factor (NGF) production.

- Injections to neuromata of local anaesthetic can have effects outlasting the pharmacological duration of local anaesthetic.
- Colchicine and vincristine both reduce the transport of NGF. They have the unfortunate effect of causing peripheral neuropathies and currently have no established role in the treatment of neuromata.
- In animal models, electrical discharge from neuromata can be decreased by noradrenaline depletion with agents such as guanethidine or bretylium.
- Topical steroids and topical glycerol suppress ectopic neural discharge in experimental neuromata.

# Chronic post-surgical pain

This refers to pain in and around the operation site. It may or may not involve the scar. It is more likely after the following surgical procedures:

- Thoracotomy.
- Coronary artery bypass grafting especially after internal mammary artery grafting.
- Sternotomy.
- Inguinal hernia repair.
- Radical neck dissection.
- Breast surgery.
- Cholecystectomy.
- Nephrectomy via flank incision.
- Pelvic surgery via Pfannensteil incision.
- Episiotomy.
- Strip of the long saphenous vein.

## Breast surgery

Studies report varying incidences of chronic pain following breast surgery, usually around 30%. It is sometimes referred to as post-mastectomy pain syndrome even if there has been no mastectomy but only wide local excision. Surgery can vary from wide local excision to radical reconstructive surgery. There are reports of pain persisting for up to 12 years. It is important to exclude recurrent disease as a cause of pain. Pain may be of different causes and more than one cause may co-exist in the same patient. To highlight the cause allows more specifically directed treatment. Further axillary node clearance and radiotherapy may contribute to the pain amalgam. The role of preservation of the intercostobrachial nerve is debated.

## Causes of pain after breast surgery

*1. Recurrent cancer.* Patients should remain under the follow-up care of an oncologist or breast surgeon whilst they have persistent pain.

*2. Radiation induced pain.* This can be the result of changes in nerve, fat, connective tissue or bone causing oedema, fibrosis, necrosis and ischaemia, or a radiation-induced brachial plexopathy. The description can give an idea as to whether the pain is likely to be nociceptive or neuropathic. Brachial plexopathy has become less common as radiotherapy techniques have improved. It develops late into disease. It is caused by loss of myelin and ischaemia. It presents as pain in the C5/C6 distribution of the treated side and with wasting and weakness of the small muscles of the hand.

**3. Post-mastectomy pain syndrome.** Neuromata should be excluded. This is a neuropathic pain syndrome but there may be associated nociceptive pain. There may be a sensation of 'phantom breast'. It presents as pain in the axilla, medial upper arm, anterior chest wall or lateral chest wall. There may be associated paraesthesiae, and allodynia is present in 20% 1 month after surgery.

**4. Associated conditions.** Frozen shoulder, carpal tunnel syndrome and lymphoedema. The latter tends only to be painful if the limb is grossly swollen and heavy or if there is a cellulitis.

An attempt to diagnose pain is helpful but in reality a symptom-orientated approach is used, dividing pain largely into nociceptive or neuropathic categories.

## Management of pain after breast surgery

- *Tricyclic antidepressants* (at a median dose of 50 mg at night) have been shown effective in post-surgical pain.
- *NSAIDs, COXIB* and simple analgesics are appropriate where there is bone or soft tissue association.
- *Capsaicin 0.075%* is successful in the treatment of post-mastectomy pain.

## Thoracotomy

- It is estimated 50% of patients have chronic pain 2 years after surgery.
- Diagnosis of mechanism of pain is important.
- *Recurrent malignant disease* must be excluded.
- *Thoracoscopy* also causes significant long term morbidity. Pain may be non-specific neuropathic pain but can be an identified single nerve neuralgia.

## Pain following cardiac surgery

There is a recognized post-coronary artery bypass graft (CABG) pain syndrome as distinct from recurrent angina. This has been reported as having an overall incidence of 56%. It is clinically neuropathic and has a severe effect on quality of life and therefore outcome from CABG. Pain can also be experienced as a consequence of the sternotomy and the use of the internal mammary artery for graft reconstruction.

## Management

Many of these pains are neuropathic in origin and logic would dictate that tricyclic antidepressants, anticonvulsants, transcutaneous nerve stimulation and capsaicin cream would be valuable. Topiramate has been described as of use in isolated intercostal neuralgia.

## Further reading

Macrae WA. Chronic pain after surgery. *British Journal of Anesthesia*, 2001; **87:** 88–98.

## Systematic review

Zhang WY, Li Wan Po A. The effectiveness of topically applied capsaicin: a meta-analysis. *European Journal of Clinical Pharmacology*, 1994; **46:** 517–22.

## Related topics of interest

Complex regional pain syndromes (p. 67); Neuropathic pain – an overview (p. 113); Nociceptive pain – an overview (p. 117); Post-amputation pain (p. 130); Sympathetic nervous system and pain (p. 153).

# SPINAL CORD INJURY

*Andrew Severn, Paul Eldridge*

Pain is a common symptom in patients with spinal cord injuries and contributes significantly to the morbidity of the condition. In some studies, it has been the pain, rather than the paraplegia, which has been the reason for inability to work. Pain may be nociceptive or neuropathic, related to the disability or the injury.

## Pathophysiology

The physiology of pain sensation after spinal cord injury has to explain the varied and distressing syndromes that are observed. The clinical picture may be confused by the presence of an incomplete lesion, or a second lesion at a lower segment of the cord.

Traditional neuroanatomy has described the effects of partial spinal cord section: in the Brown–Sequard syndrome, selective modalities are lost because the spinothalamic pathway (temperature and pain) crosses the midline near the level of the spinal root and the dorsal column (proprioception and mechanoreceptor) does not. Similarly, the development of a syrinx, a cystic lesion within the spinal cord, has its own symptomatology, which can be explained by reference to nerve pathways.

Explanations based on gross anatomical findings do not, however, explain other phenomena. Central pain syndromes occur even in the absence of a spinal cord. They can be extraordinarily complicated in their presentation, with the patient 'experiencing' not only pain, but movement and related phenomena, such as fatigue. Inhibition of modulating descending pathways accounts for some, but not all, of the increased activity of dorsal horn neurones immediately above the level of injury. In an animal experimental spinal cord preparation, abnormal activity in visceral afferents to non-noxious stimulation is due to this mechanism, and may be responsible for the exaggerated cardiovascular response that is seen with bladder distension and catheterization. Dorsal horn sensitization by nerve damage and continuing nociceptive stimulation may account for some of the changes.

## Clinical features

The spinally injured patient may present with a complete or incomplete lesion. Careful evaluation will sometimes reveal a second lesion at a lower level of the cord than the primary lesion. This may be the site of specific symptoms that would confuse the unwary. There are thus many ways in which the spinally injured patient can present.

Nociceptive pain may be overlooked as a cause of pain, unless there is an obvious other injury to account for it. The assumption that nociceptive pain will not be experienced distal to a spinal cord lesion is a dangerous one, for it fails to consider the situation with an incomplete lesion, and the effect of central disinhibition of nerve pathways which enter the cord above the level of the lesion. The causes of nociceptive pain include:

- Soft tissue trauma.
- Spinal fractures.
- Mechanical instability of the spine.
- Osteoporotic vertebral collapse.
- Pressure areas.
- Overuse of upper limbs to compensate for disability.
- Painful muscle spasm.

Neuropathic pain presents as segmental pain at the level of injury, with an area of hyperalgesia at the boundary between normal and abnormal sensation. The level of lesion is rarely precise and subtle differences in modality loss may be detected for several segments above the clinical level of the lesion. Rarely, changes of a type I complex regional pain syndrome (CRPS I) may be apparent in the dermatomal distribution corresponding to the site of the lesion. In the case of an incomplete lesion, a root lesion at a lower level may be symptomatic.

Causes of neuropathic pain include:

- Spinal cord damage.
- Compression of nerve roots.
- Compression of spinal cord by bone fragments, haematoma and scar tissue.
- Syrinx development within the spinal cord.
- Changes within the brain itself (central pain).

Central pain is of insidious onset and may occur weeks to months after the injury. Central pain may have a visceral quality. It is experienced as a burning sensation below the level of the lesion, though poorly localized, and alterations of pain and temperature sensitivity (indicative of spinothalamic tract involvement) are noticed on examination.

## Management

Treatment of pain after spinal injury requires accurate diagnosis as to the cause of the pain. Abdominal causes should be excluded before the pain is assumed to be of central origin. Visceral stimulation, either by abdominal pathology or physiological processes is dangerous when the spinal cord injury has removed the inhibitory influence on spinal reflexes. It can lead to fatal hypertension or arrhythmias.

With the exception of selective destruction of the dorsal root entry zone (DREZ lesion) for intractable segmental pain, procedures to destroy nerves are inappropriate. Surgical removal of the diseased spinal cord may result in central pain, and less drastic destruction procedures prevent the patient taking advantage of future surgical advances. Spinal decompression and stabilization is appropriate in some cases, and prevents further injury to the cord. Counter-stimulation techniques (transcutaneous electrical nerve stimulation and spinal cord stimulation) can be used when dorsal column nerve tracts remain intact.

Patients with spinal cord injury may be taking many medications and it is difficult to establish what is the specific contribution of any particular drug. However, the scheme below offers a rationale for treatment, with the evidence available summarized:

- *Tricyclic antidepressants* are valuable in many neuropathic pain states and should be considered in the management of the neuropathic pain of spinal cord injury.
- *Anticonvulsants* are valuable in many neuropathic pain states and should be considered in the management of the neuropathic pain after spinal cord injury. Gabapentin has been shown to reduce spasticity and improve the quality of life of patients with spinal cord injury, at least when used in combination with other drugs.
- *Baclofen* has been shown to reduce painful spasticity. It can be administered by the intrathecal route.
- *Opioids.* They may be worth a therapeutic trial, and have been reported to be successful in some patients.

General and psychological support for the victim of spinal injury has a role to play in preventing the morbidity of chronic pain. Pain relief has in the past received relatively little attention, and the low frequency of reports of pain has been said to be due to patients and carers adopting a stoical attitude to an inexplicable and untreatable complication.

## Related topics of interest

Multiple sclerosis (p. 91); Neuropathic pain – an overview (p. 113); Stroke (p. 150).

# STROKE

*Andrew Severn, Kate Grady*

A number of mechanisms may be responsible for the pain experienced by the victim of a stroke. Associated neurological impairment may make it difficult for pain relief to be obtained by changing position, and expressive difficulty may result in the patient suffering silently. Interpretation of complaints may be made more difficult by the emotional lability and depression encountered in some patients. Although the term 'thalamic pain' referring to a specific lesion in the central nervous system (CNS) was first used in 1906, it is clear that lesions in any part of the central nervous system can result in neuropathic pain. The term central post-stroke pain (CPSP) is therefore more appropriate. However it is also very important to realize that stroke victims also experience nociceptive pain as a consequence of postural abnormalities, spasm, contractures and pressure areas, and it may be premature to conclude an automatic diagnosis of CPSP just because of the history of stroke. Pain arising from these other causes needs specific treatment.

## Central post-stroke pain

### Pathology

Any lesion of CNS can be implicated as the cause of central pain. No single area has to be involved and there are no patterns of symptoms pertaining to any particular lesion. Pain can be experienced after haemorrhagic or thrombotic/embolic stroke. Loss of afferent input causes neuronal hyperpolarization and increased burst firing. Hyperpolarization of neurones normally involved in nociception signals the sensation of pain. Abnormal burst firing is influenced by the activity of several neurotransmitters including serotonin, noradrenaline, glutamate, γ-amino butyric acid (GABA) and histamine.

### Clinical features

There are many features, and the diagnosis cannnot be confirmed from the description alone. Most commonly it is described as burning, aching, lancinating, pricking, lacerating or pressing. There may be a background of pain which is constant or intermittent with added paroxysms of pain. It can be deep or superficial or both. It may be localized, for example to the hand or even only one side of the hand, or it may cover large areas such as the whole of the right or left side or the lower half of the body. Patients find it relatively easy to define the extent of the area of their pain. The development of pain cannot be prevented. It may occur immediately or be noticed only several months after the stroke. Autonomic changes may also be noticed. Concomitant depression or distress may compound the presentation. The diagnosis of central post-stroke pain has as a prerequisite the presence of a partial sensory loss. Allodynia and hyperalgesia also define the syndrome, being present in up to 75% of sufferers but are not essential for its diagnosis.

## Management

Alternative diagnosis should be sought and excluded. Examples are the common phenomenon of shoulder pain that affects up to 25% of patients within 2 weeks, and pains related to posture, spasticity or immobility. With the proviso that these conditions, which may lend themselves to simple specific mobilization procedures or alterations to nursing routine have been excluded, the following drugs and techniques may have a place in management.

*1. Antidepressants.* A single controlled study has estimated the NNT for anti-depressants for pain after stroke to be 1.7. These drugs are thus considered first-line treatments. There is precedent from other studies of neuropathic pain for using the tricyclic antidepressants, but there is some evidence to support the use of chlorim-ipramine as opposed to nortryptiline. In the population, predominantly elderly, under consideration, however, the anticholinergic actions of tricyclic drugs such as amitriptyline may have undesirable side-effects on cognitive functioning.

*2. Anticonvulsants.* Sodium valproate, phenytoin and carbamazepine have been claimed to be of benefit, but the latter has not withstood the scrutiny of con-trolled trial. Gabapentin, a drug that has been shown to be of benefit in painful spasticity in multiple sclerosis, has been used with effect in post-stroke pain.

*3. Antiarrhythmic drugs.* Patients who have failed to respond to adrenergic tricyclic antidepressant drugs have been reported to respond to mexiletine. Unless precluded by dizziness and nausea, dosage is 400 mg stat, 200 mg 6-hourly for 3 days, thereafter 200 mg b.d. or t.d.s.

Other treatments variously described include oral ketamine, transcutaneous nerve stimulation and spinal cord stimulation. A further development of stimula-tion technique is motor cortex stimulation, in which electrodes are implanted dur-ing craniotomy. This has been reported to be of value in some face and shoulder pains following stroke. Attempts to improve circulatory abnormalities with sympathectomy or vasodilators such as nifedipine have also been reported.

# Postural abnormalities and spasm

Shoulder pain may result from glenohumeral subluxation, and strategies designed to improve the range of movement and function of the glenohumeral joint may be valuable. These may include surface electrical stimulation, which has been shown to improve the range of passive lateral rotation of the humerus. Some patients may develop refractory pain and movement limitation for which more vigorous attempts at passive mobilization are required. Botulinum toxin has been reported of value for the relief of spasm. The overall rehabilitation of the patient, however, including the psychological well being, is important in managing the pain. Strategies for positioning and movement taught by a physiotherapist with experience in the field may obviate the need for drug treatment. Local anaesthetic block may provide short-term relief of pain and spasm and allow active and passive movement around joints to be undertaken.

# Further reading

Jensen TS, Lenz FA. Central post-stroke pain: a challenge for the scientist and clinician. *Pain*, 1995; **61:** 161–4.

# Related topics of interest

# SYMPATHETIC NERVOUS SYSTEM AND PAIN

*Kate Grady, Andrew Severn*

Peripheral nociceptor activity causes an increase in efferent sympathetic discharge, but under normal circumstances, sympathetic activity has no impact on the discharge of nociceptive neurons.

Although there is some debate as to the usefulness of such a distinction, when nociceptors appear to be under the influence of the sympathetic nervous system, pain is described as sympathetically maintained pain (SMP). When nociception is unaffected by the sympathetic nervous system the pain is described as sympathetically independent (SIP). The sympathetic nervous system may be involved in pain at any part of the neuraxis. Sympathetic nerve blocks may affect pain if it has a sympathetic component. Noradrenergically active drugs applied to the periphery, the spinal cord or centrally affect pain which has a sympathetic component. Some neuropathic pain and some cases of CRPS are sympathetically maintained. CRPS has signs directly associated with the sympathetic nervous system and is a more complex clinical picture than simply a sympathetically maintained neuropathic pain.

## Mechanisms

The mechanisms for pain which responds to sympathetic nerve blockade are:

- peripheral nociceptors which are sensitive to noradrenaline;
- sympathetic efferent activity producing low-grade ongoing activity in nociceptors;
- sprouting of sympathetic nerve fibres in dorsal root ganglia;
- the stimulation of $\alpha$ receptors in the dorsal horn;
- the altered levels of centrally acting monoamines.

## Diagnosis

A diagnosis of SMP is made by response to various manipulations of the sympathetic nervous system.

*1.  The intravenous phentolamine test.*  Phentolamine is an $\alpha_1$ and $\alpha_2$ adrenergic antagonist. It prevents excitation of noradrenaline sensitive nociceptors. Phentolamine in normal saline (30 mg 100 ml$^{-1}$) is infused over 20 min. If pain is relieved it is believed that the pain is sympathetically maintained.

*2.  Sympathetic local anaesthetic blocks*  by preventing efferent sympathetic activity also allow an assessment of the place of the sympathetic nervous system in the maintenance of the pain. Although local anaesthetics preferentially block preganglionic sympathetic fibres, false-positive results can be produced by blocking nociceptive afferents but sensory testing will alert to this.

*3.  Intravenous regional sympathetic blockade*  using a guanethidine tourniquet technique helps diagnosis. Guanethidine in normal saline (10–20 mg/20–50 ml) is injected into a limb which has been exsanguinated and to which a tourniquet has been applied. The technique has been adapted by some to inject guanethidine in a prilocaine solution to enhance patient comfort during the procedure.

**4.  Sympathomimetic drugs.**   SMP can be provoked by sympathomimetic drugs.

## Treatments

**1.  Intravenous regional sympathetic blockade.**   This technique is widely used for the treatment of sympathetically maintained pain. It comprises the injection of guanethidine to an exsanguinated limb, isolated by a tourniquet. Systematic review has failed to show difference in the treatment of complex regional pain syndrome between guanethidine and placebo. Despite this conclusion, and the suggestion leading from this, that the technique is of little value, intravenous guanethidine sympathetic block is commonly performed, and its use is believed to be justified by the past success of uncontrolled trials. It is suggested that the technique may work as a consequence of the tourniquet causing differential nerve blockade as a result of pressure and ischaemia. Guanethidine displaces noradrenaline from nerve endings. When it is used in intravenous regional sympathetic blockade, pain can transiently worsen as displacement initially increases circulating amounts of noradrenaline. Allodynia has been demonstrated during the block. The worsening of pain and the allodynia can be protected against by adding prilocaine to guanethidine for injection. Guanethidine is also available in tablet form.

**2.  Clonidine.**   Clonidine is an $\alpha_2$ adrenergic agonist. Experimentally and clinically it has been shown to have an antinociceptive effect. It is effective in treating sympathetically maintained pain. The understanding of its mechanism suggests a further role in the treatment of noradrenaline-sensitive neuromata.

Clonidine has a spinal and supraspinal action. It inhibits the release of noradrenaline from primary afferents both in the dorsal horn and at higher centres. This is a presynaptic $\alpha_2$ action. Clonidine also effects cholinergic transmission and inhibits acetylcholinesterase.

Clonidine is available as an oral preparation, and used at doses of 50–150 µg t.d.s. The absence of neurotoxicity allows intrathecal and epidural use. Used in this way it is valuable for the treatment of cancer pain when opioids are ineffective or the patient is troubled by side-effects of opioids.

Consistent with the mechanism of its main use the treatment of hypertension, clonidine causes hypotension. Rebound hypertension can occur if treatment is suddenly stopped. Bradycardia occurs. Sedation, anticholinergic effects and respiratory depression can occur.

Tizanidine has $\alpha_2$ agonist action. It is used mainly for its antispastic (useful in stump jactitation) effects but may be useful where a myofascial and neuropathic process co-exist. Dose recommendations are 2–24 mg daily in 3–4 divided doses. It does however have very sedating effects and may be best taken as a single night-time dose.

**3.  Adrenergic β-antagonists.**   Propranolol, a $\beta_2$ antagonist has been reported effective in phantom limb pain and painful diabetic neuropathy.

**4. Neuroleptic drugs.** These work through post-synaptic α blockade. Although their use is not common they have been reported to be of use as single preparations and in combination use with amitriptyline.

## Further reading

Dickenson E. Spinal cord pharmacology of pain. *British Journal of Anaesthesia*, 1995; **75**: 193–200.
Glynn C, Dawson D, Sanders R. A double-blind comparison between epidural morphine and epidural clonidine in patients with chronic non-cancer pain. *Pain*, 1988; **34**: 123–8.

## Systematic review

Jadad AR, Carroll D, Glynn CJ, McQuay HJ. Intravenous regional sympathetic blockade for pain relief in reflex sympathetic dystrophy: a systematic review and a randomised, double-blind crossover study. *Journal of Pain and Symptom Management*, 1995; **10**(1): 13–20.

## Related topics of interest

Cancer – intrathecal and epidural infusions (p. 49); Neuropathic pain – an overview (p. 113); Nociceptive pain – an overview (p. 117).

# THERAPY – ANTIARRHYTHMICS

*Kate Grady*

Neuropathic pain is caused by repetitive firing in afferent fibres which depends on influx and efflux of sodium through sodium channels. Drugs which block sodium channels can give relief from some neuropathic pains. Sodium channels are blocked by some anticonvulsants and some antiarrhythmics. Anticonvulsants are considered in their own chapter.

The antiarrhythmics most commonly considered are intravenous or intranasal lignocaine, mexiletine, tocainamide and flecanide although none of these are licensed for the treatment of pain. Mexiletine and tocainamide, by their action can be considered as systemic local anaesthetics.

A systematic review of intravenous, intranasal lignocaine, oral mexiletine and oral tocainamide in peripheral nerve injury, diabetic neuropathy, post-herpetic neuralgia, trigeminal neuralgia and pain after spinal cord injury has shown these drugs to be effective.

## Lignocaine

Lignocaine has been shown to be effective in peripheral nerve damage, post-herpetic neuralgia and painful diabetic neuropathy, but not in cancer-related pain. The best documented effective dose was 5 mg kg$^{-1}$, and when infused over 30 min was well tolerated. Adverse effects of lightheadedness and nausea and the possibility of cardiac arrhythmias must be considered. They should not be used in patients taking other antiarrhythmics and tricyclic antidepressants should be stopped.

The longer-term effects of intravenous lignocaine have not been considered although one randomized controlled trial noted a significant effect lasting up to 8 days. There is no evidence for the longer-term efficacy or safety. Currently there is no method of longer administation than prolonged infusion. It is anticipated that a lignocaine patch will become available.

Intranasal lignocaine (20–80 mg) has been shown to provide significantly better pain relief than saline.

## Mexiletine

There is no evidence for the commonly held belief that response to intravenous lignocaine is predictive of response to mexiletine. Oral mexiletine 750 mg daily was effective in two out of four randomized controlled trials. It has also been shown to be effective in HIV-induced peripheral neuropathy.

Two trials have shown it to be effective in painful diabetic neuropathy but another study shows it to have a NNT of 10.

Pain due to peripheral nerve damage is said to respond, but pain due to spinal cord injury is said not to respond.

At moderate doses for neuropathic pain, 675 mg daily up to 50% of patients developed side-effects of nausea, vomiting, abdominal pain, dizziness, headache and tremor.

Mexilitine should be started at 100–200 mg daily in divided doses and increased slowly.

**Tocainamide**

Tocainamide has been shown to be comparable to carbamezepine in trigeminal neuralgia. It has been reported to have caused serious haematological side effects.

## Systematic review

Kalso E, Tramer MR, McQuay HJ, Moore RA. Systemic local anaesthetic type drugs in chronic pain: a systematic review. *European Journal of Pain*, 1998; **2**: 3–14.

## Related topics of interest

Neuropathic pain – an overview (p. 113); Therapy – anticonvulsants (p. 158).

# THERAPY – ANTICONVULSANTS

*Kate Grady*

Neuropathic pain is caused by repetitive firing in afferent fibres. This depends on influx and efflux of sodium through sodium channels. Drugs which block sodium channels can give relief from some neuropathic pains. Sodium channels are blocked by some anticonvulsants.

The mainstay of pharmacological treatment of neuropathic pain are the antidepressants and the anticonvulsants. These drugs alleviate pain but do not treat the whole chronic pain problem. A multidisciplinary approach to non-pharmacological and behavioural methods is required. Evidence from randomized controlled trials supports the use of anticonvulsants in painful diabetic neuropathy and post-herpetic neuralgia. The effect on specific features of neuropathic pain, namely allodynia and hyperalgesia have been used as indicators of efficacy. Neuropathic pain syndromes may present with various clinical subtypes, depending on the severity of the nerve injury and the extent to which the central nervous system has become sensitized. Subtypes can be described with reference to the effectiveness of different therapies in the condition. Anticonvulsants act by membrane stabilization. Although empirical advice, based on the pathophysiology described above, has traditionally been that anticonvulsants are first-line treatment for 'lancinating' or 'stabbing' sensations associated with neuropathy, there is evidence in favour of reserving their use as second-line treatments after antidepressants for all symptoms. Significant differences between the efficacy of gabapentin and amitriptyline have not been demonstrated. Anticonvulsants are useful in combination with tricyclic antidepressants to spare increases in dose and consequent side-effects. A systematic review of the use of anticonvulsants for diabetic neuropathy and post-herpetic neuralgia offered no evidence that gabapentin is any better then other anticonvulsants.

Carbamazepine has been shown to relieve pain of trigeminal neuralgia to maximum doses of 600–2040 mg daily and given for 5–14 days. In doses of 600 mg daily for 2 weeks it has been shown to reduce the pain of diabetic neuropathy. It is started at low dose 100 mg o.d.–b.d.; a common dose is 200 mg t.d.s.–q.d.s.

Phenytoin 300 mg daily for 2 weeks has been shown to be effective in pain of diabetic neuropathy. Unwanted troublesome side-effects are common with carbamazepine and phenytoin.

Gabapentin has an unknown mechanism of action. Its effectiveness has been demonstrated in randomized controlled trials of painful diabetic neuropathy and post-herpetic neuralgia. Both pain and its physical consequences such as sleep disturbance were improved. The NNT for gabapentin is 3.2 for post-herpetic neuralgia and 3.7 for painful diabetic neuropathy. Effectiveness is claimed for the treatment of neuropathic pain in trigeminal neuralgia, complex regional pain syndromes, multiple sclerosis, neuropathic cancer pain and neuropathic back pain. The dose recommendations are to reach a range of 0.9–1.8 g daily by a daily dose increase of 300 mg. Dose escalation can be problematic and limited by side-effects of drowsiness and dizziness (in up to 25%). Ataxia, a more disabling side-effect can be a problem, but gabapentin has fewer toxic effects than carbamazepine and phenytoin. It has no known drug interactions. Cost is an issue.

Lamotrigine has been shown to relieve trigeminal neuralgia when titrated to 400 mg a day over 4 days. It has also been shown to relieve the pain of peripheral neuropathy secondary to HIV when titrated slowly to 300 mg daily. Rash is relatively common and more severe skin reactions can occur but tend to be at inappropriately high doses. Dose titration to an effective level needs to be undertaken cautiously.

Topiramate has been shown to be effective in painful diabetic neuropathy, starting at a dose of 25 mg o.d. increasing to 200 mg b.d. over a 2-week period. Its effectiveness is also claimed in mixed neuropathic pain, in which pain was improved at a mean dose of 214 mg per day (weekly titration of 25–50 mg is suggested), post-thoracotomy pain at a dose of 50 mg mane and 75 mg nocte, and trigeminal neuralgia secondary to multiple sclerosis at a dose of 150 mg per day. Fatigue and weight loss are significant side-effects.

Carbamazepine and phenytoin are licensed for use in trigeminal neuralgia. Gabapentin is licensed for the treatment of neuropathic pain of any cause.

## Systematic reviews

Collins SL, Moore RA, McQuay HJ, Wiffen P. Antidepressants and anticonvulsants for diabetic neuropathy and post-herpetic neuralgia: a quantitative systematic review. *Journal of Pain and Symptom Management*, 2000; **20**(6): 449–58.

McQuay H, Carroll D, Jadad AR, Wiffen P, Moore A. Anticonvulsant drugs for management of pain: a systematic review. *British Medical Journal*, 1995; **311**: 1047–52.

Wiffen P, Collins S, McQuay H, Carroll D, Jadad A, Moore A. *Anticonvulsant drugs for acute and chronic pain (Cochrane review)*. In: The Cochrane library, Issue 3, 2000, Oxford, Update software.

## Related topic of interest

Therapy – antidepressants (p. 160).

# THERAPY – ANTIDEPRESSANTS

*Kate Grady*

The mainstay of pharmacological treatment of neuropathic pain are the antidepressants and the anticonvulsants. These drugs alleviate pain but do not treat the whole pain problem. A multidisciplinary approach to non-pharmacological and behavioural methods may be required.

A systematic review of 21 studies, looking at ten different antidepressants in several painful syndromes showed 30% will have >50% pain relief. The overall NNT is 2.9, with NNT of 2.4 for painful diabetic neuropathy, 2.3 for post-herpetic neuralgia and 2.5 for peripheral nerve injury and central pain. Although all types of antidepressants have been suggested for use in the treatment of neuropathic pain, tricyclic drugs are more efficient than heterocyclic drugs. There is no evidence that any one tricyclic drug is better than another but side-effects may influence choice. Thus nortriptyline is frequently preferred to amitriptyline because it has less anticholinergic effects, such as dry mouth, sedation and constipation.

Analgesic effect has been shown to be independent of the effect on mood. However additional benefit may be accrued from the effect of antidepressants on the reactive component of pain. There is evidence that patients with a substantial physical basis for their back pain responded to desipramine as well as patients who did not have a physical basis. In addition systematic reviews make the following observations:

- Analgesic effect is not significantly different for pain with an organic or psychological basis.
- Analgesic effect is not significantly different in the presence or absence of depression.
- Analgesic effect is not significantly different in doses smaller than those usually effective in treating depression and in normal doses.
- Antidepressants which inhibit monoamines less selectively are more effective than selective drugs, indicating that noradrenaline and serotonin are both involved in the mechanism of pain.

The role of antidepressants in the management of low back pain is controversial. On the one hand pain relief is not consistently obtained. On the other hand associated symptoms and functional ability may be improved.

## Tricyclic antidepressants

The commonly used tricyclic antidepressants (TCA) are nortriptyline, amitriptyline, dothiepin, and imipramine. Analgesic response occurs much faster (within 4 days) than antidepressant response. TCA prevent the reuptake of endogenous noradrenaline and serotonin. Serotonin and noradrenaline within the CNS enhance the action of the descending inhibitory neural pathways at spinal cord level. To spare anticholinergic side-effects such as drowsiness and dry mouth, small doses of nortryptyline and amitriptyline such as 10 mg o.n. in the elderly or 25 mg o.n. in the more robust or imipramine 25–50 mg b.d. are used. Patients should be encouraged that side-effects reduce over time. As side-effects allow, dose can be increased at weekly intervals to achieve further therapeutic effect. Sedating antidepressants should be considered if there are problems of sleep disturbance.

## Selective serotonin reuptake inhibitors

Selective serotonin reuptake inhibitors (SSRI) have been demonstrated to work in the treatment of chronic pain, but research and experience of them is limited. Paroxetine 40 mg daily has been used to treat painful diabetic neuropathy; however, systematic review suggests NNT for paroxetine of 6.7, which compares unfavourably with the demonstrated efficacy of a susbstantial dose of imipramine with NNT of 1.4 and other TCAs at 2.4. Paroxetine and mianserin have been shown to be less effective than impipramine in various painful conditions.

Notwithstanding the comments made above about efficacy, fluoxetine and paroxetine have been shown to have a lower incidence of side-effects than tricyclic antidepressants. They may have a role where the tricyclics can not be tolerated. A systematic review recommends non-selective antidepressants to be used for depressed patients with pain complaints if antidepressants are a suitable treatment for the depression, for patients with pain of organic basis where other treatments have failed and for patients with chronic pain in the head region. It is important for the sake of the patient's self confidence and the relationship with the doctor that the patient is aware he has been prescribed an antidepressant, albeit for a different indication.

The role of the newer groups of antidepressants in chronic pain has not been established.

## Systematic reviews

McQuay HJ, Tramer M, Nye BA, Carroll D, Wiffen PJ, Moore RA. Systematic review of antidepressants in neuropathic pain. *Pain*, 1996; **68:** 217–27.

Onghena P, Van Houdenhove B. Antidepressant induced analgesia in chronic non-malignant pain: a meta analysis of 39 placebo controlled studies. *Pain*, 1992; **49**(2): 205–19.

Volmink J, Lancaster T, Gray S, Silagy C. Treatments of post herpetic neuralgia; A systematic review of randomised controlled trials. *Family Practitioner*, 1996; **13:** 84–91.

## Related topics of interest

Depression and pain (p. 73); Neuropathic pain – an overview (p. 113); Post-herpetic neuralgia (p. 133).

# THERAPY – ANTI-INFLAMMATORY DRUGS

*Kate Grady*

There are two classes of anti-inflammatory drugs that will be considered here. These are the non-steroidal anti-inflammatory drugs (NSAIDs) and the cyclo-oxygenase type 2 inhibitor drugs (COXIBs).

Both work by reduction of prostaglandin synthesis, a marker of the inflammatory response and a potent compound in inducing sensitization of primary afferent nociceptors. They differ in the degree to which they selectively inhibit each of two isozymes of cyclo-oxygenase, known as type 1 and type 2. Type 1 enzyme is present in tissue during health, whereas type 2 is induced as a consequence of tissue damage. Selective inhibition of the type 2 isozyme is therefore a logical target for therapeutic action and a higher therapeutic ratio. The gastrointestinal side effects of NSAIDs are a consequence of type 1 inhibition.

NSAIDs inhibit both isozymes, whereas COXIBs have a dose-dependent selective action on the type 2 isozyme. Etodolac and meloxicam are preferential type 2 inhibitors with actions on the type 1 isozyme at therapeutic doses. The expected improvement in gastrointestinal side effects has been demonstrated in trials comparing meloxicam with NSAIDs. Rofecoxib and celecoxib are selective inhibitors of the type 2 isozyme. Further COXIBs, parecoxib and valdecoxib, are under development.

Each year 0.5–2% of those taking NSAIDs have a serious gastrointestinal event. The risks of adverse events has been shown to be greater in the elderly and those with a history of ulcer, gastrointestinal bleeding, cardiovascular disease, or if taking steroids or anticoagulants. The rationale for the use of COXIBs is a preservation of the type 1 isozyme with a reduction in gastrointestinal complications.

## Use and efficacy

### NSAIDs

NSAIDs should be given at the lowest effective dose and the need should be reviewed regularly. Failure to respond to one drug does not imply failure to respond to another. Different drugs of the group should be tried. Choice of drug within this category is influenced by side-effect profile. Ibuprofen has a low incidence (5–15%) of gastrointestinal effects and is a useful first choice as 200–800 mg t.d.s. Diclofenac, as 50 mg t.d.s., has a higher incidence of gastric side-effects (up to 25%). Systematic review has demonstrated that tenoxicam is better tolerated than indomethacin. Gastric protection (with misoprostol or proton pump inhibitor) should be considered in those at risk of gastrointestinal complications. Misoprostol protects against gastrointestinal side-effects and is available as a combination preparation with NSAIDs. The decision to use NSAIDs should be influenced by a view about the likelihood of inflammation. The use of NSAIDs in osteo-arthritis, a chronic condition in which there is little evidence of inflammation, is controversial.

## COXIBs

Rofecoxib is licensed for pain relief in osteoarthritis but not rheumatoid arthritis. 12.5 mg once daily is recommended, increasing to a maximum of 25 mg daily. The increased dose should be used cautiously in older patients. It has been shown at a dose of 12.5–25 mg daily to be equally as effective in pain relief in osteoarthritis as ibuprofen 800 mg t.d.s. and diclofenac 50 mg t.d.s. It has been shown to be superior to placebo in rheumatoid arthritis at a dose of 25–50 mg daily.

Celecoxib is licensed for pain relief in both osteoarthritis and rheumatoid arthritis in doses between 100 and 200 mg b.d.

Celecoxib relieves the pain of osteoarthritis of the knee at doses of 200 mg a day (single or divided doses). Celecoxib 100 or 200 mg b.d. and naproxen 500 mg b.d. were equally effective in improving joint pain and function. Pharmacokinetic studies suggest that the initial dose should be lower in the elderly and Afrocaribbean patients.

In rheumatoid arthritis celecoxib has been shown to be effective as an anti-inflammatory and an analgesic at a dose of 100–400 mg b.d. Celecoxib 100 mg, 200 mg or 400 mg b.d. has been shown to be similarly as effective as naproxen 500 mg b.d. in reducing joint pain and swelling, and as effective at a dose of 200 mg b.d. as diclofenac 75 mg b.d.

# Unwanted effects

## Gastrointestinal

**1. Rofecoxib versus NSAID.** For rofecoxib at 12.5–25 mg daily the incidence of epigastric discomfort, heartburn, nausea and diarrhoea is not different significantly from ibuprofen 2.4 g daily or diclofenac 150 mg daily. However the incidence of endoscopic ulcer diagnosis appears to be reduced when rofecoxib 25–50 mg daily is compared with ibuprofen 800 mg t.d.s., and is not significantly higher than that seen after placebo administration over a 12-week period of observation. In patients with a prior history of peptic ulceration, the incidence of serious complications has not been shown to be reduced.

**2. Celecoxib versus NSAID.** Systematic review from meta-analysis suggests there may be a significantly lower incidence of abdominal pain, dyspepsia and nausea with celecoxib 50, 100, 200 and 400 mg twice daily than with naproxen 500 mg twice daily. In a study comparing celecoxib 400 mg twice daily with diclofenac 75 mg twice daily or ibuprofen 800 mg t.d.s. on the incidence of confirmed ulcer complications, the incidence was significantly lower with celecoxib than the others.

A study of 32 healthy volunteers showed six developed an endoscopically detected gastric ulcer after one week's treatment with naproxen 500 mg b.d. while no ulcer developed with celecoxib 100 mg b.d. or 200 mg b.d. Other studies have shown the incidence of duodenal ulceration to be lower with celecoxib (100–400 mg b.d.) than with NSAIDs (naproxen 500 mg b.d. and diclofenac 75 mg b.d.). A pooled analysis of 14 RCTs showed the incidence of ulcer complications with celecoxib 25–400 mg b.d. to be eight times lower than NSAIDs and similar to that in patients receiving placebo.

## Platelets

NSAIDs inhibit platelets reversibly, and should be avoided where there is a risk of provoking bleeding. Five days treatment with rofecoxib 12.5 mg or 25 mg daily or 10 days treatment with 600 mg twice daily does not inhibit platelet activity or prolong bleeding time. The concomitant use of aspirin as a platelet inhibitor in the management of arterial occlusive disease or as prophylaxis against deep venous thrombosis may negate all the potential benefits of selective COX 2 inhibition, and unmask all the problems associated with nonspecific enzyme inhibition.

## Renal effects and sodium retention

Although the COX 2 isozyme is believed to be predominantly an enzyme involved in the mechanism of inflammation, prostaglandins synthesized under the influence of the COX 2 isozyme may also have a role in homeostasis in the kidney, brain and reproductive organs. The role is not well understood.

Sodium retention and a fall in glomerular filtration rate has been shown with NSAIDs, and therapeutic doses of rofecoxib. A similar effect is claimed to occur with celecoxib. There is evidence however to show a lower incidence of hypertension or increase in serum creatinine with COXIB use than with NSAIDs.

In practice NSAIDs with gastric protection are accepted as a first-line treatment for many conditions where there is a risk of gastrointestinal complications. The value of COXIB has to be judged against this recommendation. COXIBs are found to be as effective as NSAIDs but although there is some reduction of risk of serious gastro-intestinal events the evidence of that is small. Neither NSAIDs or COXIBs should be used in patients with active ulcers or bleeding, creatinine clearance of less than 30 mlmin$^{-1}$, severe hepatic dysfunction or congestive cardiac failure. The use of either drug for the long-term maintenance of painful conditions in which inflammation plays only a small part in the overall process, such as osteoarthritis, is controversial, and not well supported by trials comparing NSAIDs against standard analgesics. Having said that, there is a suggestion that these interesting drugs have a central action on mechanisms of signalling within the spinal cord and may have their own analgesic action that is independent on the mechanisms of suppressing inflammation.

## Further reading

Bensen WG, Fiechtner JJ, McMillen JI et al. Treatment of osteoarthritis with celecoxib, a cyclooxygenase 2 inhibitor: a randomised controlled trial. Proceedings of the Mayo Clinic, 1999; **74:** 1095–1105.

Day R, Morrison B, Luza A et al for the Rofecoxib / Ibuprofen Comparator study group. A randomised trial of the efficacy and tolerability of the COX 2 inhibitor rofecoxib vs ibuprofen in patients with osteoarthritis. Archives of Internal Medicine, 2000; **160:** 1781–7.

Emery P, Zeidler H, Kvein TK et al. Celecoxib versus diclofenac in long term management of rheumatoid arthritis: randomised double blind comparison. Lancet, 1999; **354:** 2106–11.

Silverstein FE, Faich G, Goldstein GL et al. Gastrointestinal toxicity with celecoxib vs nonsteroidal anti-inflammatory drugs for osteoarthritis and rheumatoid arthritis. The CLASS study: a randomised controlled trial. JAMA, 2000; **284:** 1247–55.

## Systematic review

Goldstein JL, Silverstein FE, Agrawal NM, Hubbard RC, Kaiser J, Maurath CJ, Verburg KM, Geis GS. Reduced risk of upper gastrointestinal ulcer complications with celecoxib, a novel COX 2 inhibitor. *American Journal of Gastroenterology*, 2000; **95**: 1681–90.

## Related topics of interest

Musculoskeletal pain syndromes (p. 95); Nociceptive pain – an overview (p. 117); Osteoarthritis (p. 121).

# THERAPY – BOTULINUM TOXIN

*Kate Grady*

Botulinum toxin is licensed for the symptomatic treatment of blepharospasm and hemifacial spasm. It is used without licence to relieve pains due to other types of muscle spasm.

The pharmaceutical preparation contains botulinum toxin of the type A serotype, serum albumin and sodium chloride. The botulinum toxin was first isolated in 1895 from the food of victims of food poisoning. It was then first recognized as a neurotoxin.

## Mechanism

The neurotoxic action reduces neuromuscular transmission thereby causing skeletal muscle weakness and inhibition of muscle spasm. Botulinum toxin selectively acts on peripheral cholinergic nerve endings. It enters the nerve terminal and causes localized chemical destruction. This prevents the release of acetylcholine at the neuromuscular junction. Efficient neuromuscular transmission depends on the release of acetylcholine from the axonal terminal and its binding to the postsynaptic receptors to effect the muscle action potential. Without the synthesis and release of acetylcholine the muscle action potential is prevented. After the nerve end plate has shrivelled it starts to regenerate by sprouting. When the sprouts reach the muscle surface a new neuromuscular junction has formed. Regeneration takes approximately 3 months. When it is complete, tone and muscle spasms recur. At that stage the injection of botulinum toxin can be repeated indefinitely. Tachyphylaxis has been shown. In addition to its effects on the motor nerve ending, botulinum toxin has also been reported to have an analgesic effect.

## Pharmacokinetics

Botulinum toxin is given intramuscularly to affected peripheral muscles. Its spread is dependent on the dose of drug and the volume of diluent. It is taken up by neuronal transport to the spinal cord where it is broken down to inactive metabolites.

## Use

Botulinum toxin is available in single-patient-use vials each containing 100 units. The preparation is freeze dried. It is recommended that it be reconstituted with normal saline although workers in the USA are using local anaesthetic as solvent to enhance the speed of onset of effect. Diluted with normal saline the onset of action is at approximately 3 days and the effect peaks at 1–2 weeks after administration. Injections are sometimes carried out under electromyographic control or with the use of radio-opaque dye and fluoroscopy.

The manufacturer's recommended maximum dose in the treatment of blepharospasm is 100 units per 12 weeks. The maximum dose used by workers in the USA for the relief of other muscle spasms is 400 units per 12 weeks. The $LD_{50}$ for single use in a 70 kg person is 3000 units. Depending on the size and number of muscles needing treatment, doses as small as 1.25 units are used for blepharospasm and 30 units for painful conditions secondary to muscle spasm. Inhibition of muscle activity of 50% allows the performance of otherwise difficult physiotherapy. The physiotherapy brings further improvement in muscle function. Painful conditions in which botulinum toxin has been used include:

- Back and myofascial pain.
- Spasticity and painful contractures.
- Headache.

There is evidence of efficacy in all these conditions, but systematic reviews on the use of botulinum in spasticity do not comment specifically on pain control.

**1. *Back and myofascial pains.*** Botulinum has been shown to be effective in low back pain when injected paravertebrally at five sites, 40 units per site. Botulinum toxin has been used to treat myofascial pains of the neck, shoulder and low back. Injections have also been carried out to psoas and quadratus lumborum muscles to relieve spasticity. Muscle spasm precipitating pain in conditions such as multiple sclerosis has been treated. Pain caused by an abnormal posture forced by muscle spasm can be treated by botulinum toxin.

**2. *Spasticity and painful contractures.*** Secondary contractures resulting from neurological deficit after stroke or from disuse as in the complex regional pain syndromes (CRPS) is reported to be relieved by botulinum toxin. In cervical dystonia over 70% have pain. The injection of doses of botulinum toxin ranging from 100 to 236 units has been reported to give relief of spasm with consequent reduction in pain. In all these conditions the relief of spasticity offers an opportunity and is not an alternative to this.

**3. *Headache.*** Botulinum has been shown to be effective in the prevention of tension headache and migraine.

## Side-effects

Local muscle weakness can occur from local spread of drug. Injections into the neck may thus affect swallowing. Misplaced injections can paralyse nearby muscle groups extensively. Excessive doses may paralyse muscles distant to the site of injection. Spread is affected by both dose and volume of diluent. Generalized malaise, about which the patient should be informed, can follow the treatment.

Botulinum toxin is potent in reducing muscle spasm and although currently unlicensed for the purpose, there may be a place for it in the relief of muscle spasm which causes pain. It has been found to have few side-effects. The established regeneration of nerve makes it acceptable in terms of no long-term destructive effect. It offers a useful addition to the pain clinician's armamentarium as a drug which may relieve pain and also improve function.

## Further reading

Childers MK, Wilson DJ, Galate JF, Smith BK. Treatment of painful muscle syndromes with botulinum toxin: a review. *Journal of Back and Musculoskeletal Rehabilitation*, 1998; **10**(2): 89–96.

Raj PP. Botulinum for the treatment of pain (editorial). *Pain Digest*, 1998; **8**(6): 335–6.

Racz G. Botulinum as a new approach for refractory pain syndromes. *Pain Digest*, 1998; **8**(6): 353–6.

## Systematic review

Ade Hall RA, Moore AP. *Botulinum toxin type A in the treatment of lower limb spasticity in cerebral palsy.* In: the Cochrane Library, Issue 4, 2000, Oxford: Update software.

## Related topics of interest

Complex regional pain syndromes (p. 67); Multiple sclerosis (p. 91).

# THERAPY – CANNABINOIDS

*Kate Grady, Andrew Severn*

The cannabinoids are derived from the resin of the plant *Cannabis sativa*. The only known active constituent is 9-tetrahydrocannabinol ($\delta$9-THC). Other cannabinoids are an oral synthetic nitrogen analogue of THC and intramuscular levonantradol. There are claims for their use in nausea and vomiting, appetite stimulation in HIV-infected patients, movement disorders and glaucoma. There have also been claims that cannabinoids are useful in the treatment of migraine and painful spasticity in multiple sclerosis and spinal cord injury. There is some evidence that they are analgesic in humans. A systematic review of nine randomized controlled trials has concluded that there need to be further trials into their use in spasticity and neuropathic pain but they have no place in the management of post-operative pain. A double-blind comparison with placebo in a patient with prior history of cannabinoid use has demonstrated an opioid-sparing effect in chronic pain.

## Mechanisms of action

It is suggested from animal studies that cannabinoids reduce the behaviour believed to equate with the clinical syndromes of allodynia and hyperalgesia. From animal evidence, here summarized, it is believed that the brain is probably the site of action, but there is evidence for a spinal cord site of action.

*1. Opioid receptor agonism.* Perinatal exposure to cannabinoids results in analgesia, morphine tolerance and an abstinence syndrome when given naloxone. Naloxone and other opioid receptor antagonists, specifically the $\kappa_1$ antagonists block the antinociceptive actions of cannabinoids. They do not prevent the behavioural effects. An effect has been observed when the opioid receptor is blocked by spinal administration.

*2. Cannabinoid receptor agonism.* Cannabinoid receptors have been identified; CB1 receptors on central and peripheral neurons and CB2 receptors on immune cells. The identification and cloning of specific cannabinoid receptors has been followed by the identification of an endogenous ligand called anandamide. The function of these receptors and ligands remains unclear. Cannabinoid receptor activation reduces the amplitude of voltage-gated calcium currents, thereby decreasing excitability and neurotransmitter release. The finding of further subclasses of receptors offers potential for separating analgesic actions from the harmful psychotropic actions by the development of synthetic analogues. The spleen contains cannabinoid receptors.

*3. Prostaglandin metabolism.* Anandamide is an intermediate product of arachidonic acid metabolism. Synthetic cannabinoids have been shown to reduce arachidonic acid-induced inflammation, presumably by an action on inhibition of eicosanoid synthesis.

## Pharmacokinetics

$\delta$9-THC is highly lipid-soluble and readily absorbed from the gastrointestinal tract and lungs. Bioavailability after oral ingestion is about 6%. It has, like other lipid-soluble compounds, a large volume of distribution. It is metabolized to polar water-soluble compounds before excretion by the kidney, although intestinal elimination accounts for some of the drug.

## Clinical effects

The best that can be achieved with cannabis is an antinociceptive effect equivalent to 60 mg codeine. The anti-inflammatory effect is unlikely to be as valuable as the currently available drugs. There is inadequate evidence to support their use in the management of more complex pain. In addition to the actions described above, cannabinoids lower intraocular pressure. Inhalation of the drug is associated with carboxyhaemoglobin production, and intrauterine growth retardation and an increase in childhood leukaemia are features of the children of women who use cannabinoids in pregnancy. Central nervous system side-effects include psychomotor and cognitive impairment. Psychiatric syndromes encountered with cannabinoid use include mania, anxiety and depression, and there is a six-fold greater incidence of schizophrenia in heavy users than in non-users.

Any potential clinical benefit in the management of chronic pain must be weighed against the hazards of the drug, and the potential harm that may result from widespread availability and social acceptability if legalization were undertaken.

## Systematic review

Campbell FA, Tramer MR, Carroll D, Reynolds DJM, Moore RA, McQuay HJ. Are cannabinoids an affective and safe treatment option in the management of pain? A qualitative systematic review. *British Medical Journal*, 2001; **323:** 13.

## Further reading

Doyle E, Spence AA. Cannabis as a medicine? *British Journal of Anaesthesia*, 1995; **74:** 359–61.
Holdcroft A, Smith M, Jacklin A, Hodgson H, Smith B, Newton M, Evans F. Pain relief with oral cannabinoids in familial Mediterranean fever. *Anaesthesia*, 1997; **52:** 483–6.
Robson P. Cannabis as a medicine: Time for the Phoenix to rise? *British Medical Journal*, 1998; **316:** 1034–5.

## Related topics of interest

Multiple sclerosis (p. 91); Nociceptive pain – an overview (p. 113).

# THERAPY – CAPSAICIN

*Kate Grady*

Capsaicin is a specific chemical entity, 8-methyl-*N*-vanillyl-noneamide of the capsaicinoid family. It is licensed for the treatment of post-herpetic neuralgia and painful diabetic neuropathy at its 0.075% concentration and at 0.025% for osteoarthritis of knees.

## Mechanism of action

Capsacinoids are molecules derived from chilli peppers. There is a specific receptor for capsaicinoids called VR1. It is present only on a subpopulation of C fibres. These fibres as well as generating pain are involved in a process known as neurogenic inflammation. This is a phenomenon mediated via nerve growth factors and other chemical mesengers carried within microtubular structures of the nerve and responsible for a localized anti-inflammatory response. After initial exposure the neurones become insensitive to all other stimuli including further capsaicin. This requires that capsaicin is regularly applied to desensitize the nerve and deplete transmitters. It also works by depletion of substance P from the C fibre endings in the periphery and the dorsal horn.

## Efficacy

*1. Painful diabetic neuropathy.* Capsaicin 0.075% compares favourably with placebo in three out of five trials in the treatment of painful diabetic neuropathy. The NNT is 5.9. Another systematic review calculates the figure from pooled data from four trials as 4.2. One randomized trial has demonstrated it to be as effective as amitriptyline 25–125 mg daily in improving pain, sleep and daily activity.

*2. Post-herpetic neuralgia.* The combined NNT from two randomized controlled trials has been calculated as 5.3.

*3. Peripheral nerve injury.* The NNT is 3.5.

*4. Post-mastectomy pain.* A beneficial effect is demonstrated in a randomized controlled trial.

*5. Osteoarthritis of the knee.* Three randomized controlled trials of the 0.025% preparation over 4 weeks in 382 patients have been reviewed and a combined NNT of 3.3 has been calculated.

In addition benefit is claimed for neuropathic stump pain, neck pain, loin pain – haematuria syndrome, complex regional pain syndromes and cutaneous pain associated with tumour. Intranasal application has been reported effective in cluster headaches.

Very high concentrations of 5–10% have been used in complex regional pain syndromes and neuropathic pain. The irritant effect of such high concentrations requires that the drug is administered under regional blockade. One technique involves the application of the concentrated preparation into the ureters after catheterization at cystoscopy: epidural analgesia is required for several days.

Capsaicin is being studied for the treatment of cystitis, pain associated with human immunodeficiency virus and painful or itching cutaneous disorders from scars.

## Adverse effects

There were no serious adverse effects reported during a study looking at application for an average of 20 weeks. Stinging and burning at the application site occurs in 59% of patients but this was mainly in the first week and disappeared over the course of the study, consistent with its mechanism of action. There are anecdotal reports of attenuation of stinging and burning by the application of a local anaesthetic preparation before the capsaicin.

Studies suggest that continued application is necessary to maintain pain relief. In the author's experience relief of pain can be maintained following discontinuation of treatment.

## Systematic review

Zhang WY, Li Wan Po A. The effectiveness of topically applied capsaicin: a metanalysis. *European Journal of Clinical Pharmacology*, 1994; **46:** 517–22.

## Related topics of interest

Neuropathic pain – an overview (p. 113); Nociceptive pain – an overview (p. 117).

# THERAPY – KETAMINE AND OTHER NMDA ANTAGONISTS

*Kate Grady*

Ketamine is an anaesthetic drug with a few notable features which have resulted in its introduction to pain clinic practice. The rationale for its use is supported by animal studies which allow tentative conclusions to be drawn about a mechanism of action. However, the extrapolation of animal data, based on electrophysiological and behavioural studies, to the human experience of pain is always difficult. The evidence to support the use of ketamine in chronic pain is necessarily limited. Ketamine is valuable for its excellent analgesic properties at subanaesthetic doses, and at anaesthetic doses for its freedom from the effects of cardiovascular and pharyngeal reflex depression which characterize other anaesthetic agents. As such it has a unique place for providing analgesia and anaesthesia for environments in which other agents would be difficult to use, for example at the site of a major accident or on the battlefield. The drug is limited by major side-effects, however, notably cardiovascular stimulation, increased cerebral blood flow, and psychological disturbance. The role of the NMDA system and 'windup' in the production of a chronic pain syndrome has not been clearly elucidated. It has been shown however that subanaesthetic doses of i.v. ketamine of 0.5 mg kg$^{-1}$ bolus followed by 0.25 mg kg$^{-1}$ h$^{-1}$ reduce hyperalgesia and are an adjuvant in post-operative analgesia.

## Mechanisms of action

The animal experimental evidence for a mechanism of action includes the following.

*1.* **N-*methyl-D-aspartate receptor (NMDA) antagonism.*** NMDA receptors are believed to be involved in the spinal cord processing of nociceptive input, where they respond to excitatory amino acids released from the central processes of primary afferent nociceptors. Their activation by nociceptors is believed to result in a response, 'windup', which may outlast the duration of action of the activation impulse and stimulate the spinal cord cell to metabolic activity. Their inactivation by ketamine is suggested, but not proven, as a manoeuvre to prevent the development of a chronic pain syndrome. It is further suggested that the observed synergism between opioids and ketamine is mediated via a common action on the NMDA receptor. In animal models of neuropathic pain, ketamine appears to restore opioid responsiveness.

*2.* **Opioid receptor agonism.** Binding of ketamine to opioid receptors in central nervous system tissue has been observed.

*3.* **Serotoninergic and adrenergic mechanisms.** Synaptic uptake of serotonin and noradrenaline is inhibited, and the antinociceptive action of spinally administered ketamine can be reversed by phentolamine and serotonin receptor antagonists.

*4.* **Cholinergic mechanisms.** Physostigmine, a centrally acting anticholinesterase, can reverse the sedation and anaesthesia of ketamine, while 4-aminopyridine, an antagonist of competitive neuromuscular blockade, speeds recovery from ketamine anaesthesia.

## Pharmacokinetics

Ketamine is metabolized in the liver to an active metabolite, norketamine, which has analgesic properties, but is believed to have fewer side-effects than ketamine. In this respect, oral treatment, despite a bioavailability of only 17%, may be preferred over parenteral treatment, where the benefits of the active metabolite are not obtained.

## Pharmacodynamics

The incidence and severity of the two major side-effects are dose related. Cardiovascular side-effects include increases in heart rate, blood pressure, cardiac output, systemic vascular resistance, and pulmonary artery pressure, and can be attenuated by benzodiazepines. Their origin is in the stimulation of the central nervous system by the drug, and because of this, the drug is contraindicated in the presence of raised intracranial pressure or seizures. The psychological disturbances take the form of alterations of mood or body image, feelings of spatial disorientation, vivid dreams, hallucinations, pleasant or unpleasant illusions, and complicated emergence from anaesthesia. They can occur with the use of ketamine by infusion for analgesia. Their occurrence can be reduced by the use of slow infusion rates. Intravenous midazolam is effective in countering the side-effects observed after intravenous ketamine. This is used at doses between 2.5 and 15 mg per day, as an infusion. Alternatives are the use of oral midazolam, 0.5 mg kg$^{-1}$, or diazepam 5–10 mg. Haloperidol 2–4 mg is an alternative.

## Clinical uses

Ketamine is used in malignant and non-malignant neuropathic pain. No oral preparation is available; the parenteral preparation is given orally or sublingually. A suggested oral dose is 50 mg t.d.s. and sublingually 10 mg t.d.s. The dose can be titrated against response and side-effects.

It has been shown to reduce pain in fibromyalgia. For cancer pain, ketamine has been used for incident pain, painful cutaneous lesions, bone pain, tenesmus, and neuropathic pain, including the pain of spinal cord compression. Its use is best considered as an alternative or adjunct to opioids where they ineffective or poorly tolerated. Subcutaneous and intravenous infusions at rates of between 40 and 500 mg per 24 h have given relief: there is a wide variation in response which requires the titration of drug to achieve a response. The subcutaneous route is complicated by the presence of a skin reaction in 20% of patients, which requires regular resiting of the subcutaneous cannula.

Severe phantom limb pain and post-herpetic neuralgia have been reported to respond to parenteral ketamine. The single dose for intravenous response is reported between 0.125 and 0.3 mg kg$^{-1}$, or as an infusion at 0.2 mg kg$^{-1}$ h$^{-1}$.

Ketamine is available in a preservative-free form for epidural and intrathecal use but this should be undertaken with caution. Ketamine administered epidurally has been reported as being effective in the treatment of Complex Regional Pain Syndrome type 1.

## Other *N*-methyl D-aspartate receptor antagonists

Worldwide, the clinically available NMDA antagonists are ketamine, dextromethorphan, memantine, amantadine and three clinically used opioids which have NMDA activity, methadone, dextropropoxyphene and ketobemidone. There are reports of the success of all of these in modulating pain and hyperalgesia.

## Further reading

Idvall J. Ketamine, a review of clinical applications. *Anaesthetic Pharmacology Review*, 1995; **3:** 82–9.

Luczak J, Dickenson AH, Kotlinska-Lemieszek A. The role of ketamine, an NMDA receptor antagonist, in the management of pain. *Progress in Palliative Care*, 1995; **3:** 127–34.

Mercadante S. Ketamine in cancer pain: an update. *Palliative Medicine*, 1996; **10:** 225–30.

## Related topics of interest

Cancer – other drugs (p. 60); Neuropathic pain – an overview (p. 113); Nociceptive pain – an overview (p. 117).

# THERAPY – NERVE BLOCKS: AUTONOMIC

*Andrew Severn*

Nerve blocks of the sympathetic nervous system are indicated for the control of pain where nociceptive afferents travel with the nerves of the autonomic system, or where an effect of blockade of the efferent autonomic nervous system is required. Efferent autonomic blockade has two major effects:

- removal of the influence of catecholamines from nociceptors;
- increased blood flow.

The analgesic effects of sympathetic block can be usefully considered as direct and indirect effects. Direct effects result from the removal of a nociceptive pathway, and indirect effects from the modulation of the nociceptive pathway, such that it is less sensitive to the effects of stimulation. This mechanism may be of importance in the pathogenesis of 'sympathetically mediated pain'. Catecholamines are implicated in the process of sensitization of primary afferents in nociceptive and neuropathic pain.

The sympathetic nervous system arises from the spinal roots of the thoracic and lumbar segments. Pre-ganglionic fibres exit from the spinal nerve as the white communicating ramus and pass to ganglia on the paravertebral sympathetic chain. Some fibres pass through the ganglion as pre-ganglionic fibres and synapse in more distal ganglia, from which fibres are distributed along blood vessels. Others form synapses within the ganglion, and post-synaptic fibres form the grey communicating ramus which joins the mixed spinal nerve. Visceral afferents are not themselves technically part of the sympathetic nervous system although their fibres pass through the ganglia and can be blocked in these ganglia.

The anatomy of the sympathetic nervous system lends itself to selective nerve blockade, which can be achieved without motor or somatic sensory loss. Local anaesthetic blockade is sometimes performed as a 'diagnostic' procedure, to enable information to be obtained about the influence of the sympathetic system on the pain. Although the short-term results of sympathetic block may be successful in, for example, reducing the pain of a complex regional pain syndrome, the long-term effects of permanent nerve blockade cannot be guaranteed.

Description of sympathetic nerve blocks is described with reference to the major anatomical landmarks of the sympathetic nervous system.

## Stellate ganglion

Three cervical sympathetic ganglia are formed from the fibres which originate from the upper thoracic nerve roots. The lowest of these fuses with the first thoracic ganglion to form the stellate ganglion, which lies superficial to the prevertebral fascia overlying the prominent anterior tubercle of the sixth cervical vertebra. An anterior approach, facilitated by retracting the carotid sheath laterally is possible at this level. Local anaesthetic block results in a block of the sympathetic supply to the cerebral vasculature, the eye and the upper limb, as evidenced by a Horner's syndrome and warmth in the upper limb. Complications include accidental injection into the vertebral artery, the epidural space and the subarachnoid space. These risks require that the procedure is performed where there are facilities for resuscitation. The proximity of the recurrent laryngeal nerve and the cervical nerve roots accounts for the minor inconvenience of block of these nerves.

## Thoracic paravertebral chain

Direct approach to the thoracic sympathetic chain is complicated by the close proximity of the pleura to the chain, and the risk of pneumothorax. However, the interpleural technique of nerve block, involving the positioning of a catheter between visceral and parietal pleura affords one way of achieving block of the thoracic chain and the nerves associated with it, namely the greater, lesser and least splanchnic nerves. An alternative technique, which does not involve the needle being deliberately introduced into the pleural cavity is the thoracic paravertebral injection. In this technique, somatic and sympathetic fibres are blocked.

## Coeliac plexus

The coeliac plexus lies anterior to the aorta and surrounds the coeliac artery. It consists of three paired ganglia in which fibres from the greater, lesser and least splanchnic nerves form synapses, and through which visceral afferent fibres pass. The technique of coeliac plexus block involves the passage of needles, either side of the aorta, at the level of the body of the first lumbar vertebra, using a posterolateral approach. Needles are advanced from a point 6–7 cm from the midline under X-ray control, to a position in front of the first lumbar vertebral body. Several variations of the technique have been described, including a transaortic approach, in which the needle is passed through the aorta, transcrural and a retrocrural approach, and the use of computed tomography imaging to aid needle localization. The most notable complication, and one which limits the application of an effective technique to patients with limited life expectancy, is the development of paraplegia as a result of damage to the arterial supply to the spinal cord. This complication has been variously attributed to direct needle damage, arterial spasm, direct injection of neurolytic solution or spread of neurolytic solution. Side-effects of coeliac plexus block have been estimated as follows from pooling of data from several reports: local pain in 72%, diarrhoea in 41% and hypotension in 36%, with the incidence of more serious side-effects occurring in 3%.

## Lumbar sympathetic chain

The lumbar sympathetic chain can be interrupted where it lies in the paravertebral gutter. In this position it lies conveniently separated from the lumbar plexus by the psoas muscle. The percutaneous approach to the sympathetic chain involves passage of a needle from a position some 7–8 cm lateral to the midline. With this approach, the transverse process may not be encountered. The classical technique sought the transverse process as a landmark and then reintroduced the needle to pass to the anterior aspect of the vertebral body. Using X-ray control, a mandatory requirement, the landmark of the transverse process can be ignored. X-ray contrast should be seen to be dispersed medially when the needle is in the paravertebral gutter: lateral spread implies injection into or posterior to the psoas muscle, with the risk of damage to the lumbar plexus. The technique of lumbar sympathectomy carries with it a risk of genitofemoral neuritis that seems to be not influenced by the care that is taken to avoid depositing neurolytic solution on the genitofemoral nerve.

## Superior hypogastric plexus

The superior hypogastric plexus lies retroperitoneally at the junction of the fifth lumbar vertebra and the sacrum, and is a bilateral structure. The technique of approach is analogous to that of percutaneous block of the lumbar sympathetic chain, except that the needle is advanced caudally to pass between the transverse process of the fifth lumbar vertebra and the sacral ala. This can be very difficult to achieve, particularly as the gap between the two may be very narrow and the fifth lumbar nerve is in close proximity. Successful treatment of a variety of pelvic pain syndromes, including cancer, has been reported.

## Peripheral autonomic system

The technique of intravenous regional anaesthesia involves the use of a sympathetic system-blocking drug, such as guanethidine, being administered into a limb that is isolated from the rest of the body by a tourniquet. The tourniquet itself may have an effect on the function of the autonomic system. All local anaesthetic nerve blocks have the ability to block autonomic fibres as well as the somatic sensory and motor fibres.

## Clinical indications

Block, either with local anaesthetic or neurolytic solution of afferent nociceptive fibres is a valuable technique for the treatment of visceral pain arising from structures served by the appropriate ganglia. On the other hand, neurolytic block of efferent fibres is a more controversial subject. Block with local anaesthetic may help establish the role of the sympathetic nervous system in complex regional pain syndromes and neuropathic pain conditions such as post-herpetic neuralgia, and repeated procedures may allow for extensive rehabilitation by offering short-term pain relief at regular intervals. Block of the sympathetic nervous system is useful for the treatment of limb ischaemia and Raynaud's phenomenon.

## Further reading

Plancarte R, Amescua C, Patt RB, Aldrete A. Superior hypogastric plexus block for pelvic cancer pain. *Anesthesiology*, 1990; **73**: 236–9.

## Systematic review

Carr D, Eisenberg E, Chalmers TC. Neurolytic celiac plexus block for cancer pain – a meta analysis. In: *Proceedings of the 7th World Congress on Pain, Paris.* Seattle: IASP Press, 1993; 338.

## Related topics of interest

Cancer – nerve blocks (p. 53); Complex regional pain syndromes (p. 67); Pelvic and vulval pain (p. 125); Post-herpetic neuralgia (p. 133).

# THERAPY – NERVE BLOCKS: SOMATIC AND LESION TECHNIQUES

*Andrew Severn*

Sensory nerve blocks are widely used in chronic pain management for diagnostic and therapeutic purposes. Local anaesthetic agents and neurolytic substances such as phenol, alcohol, or glycerol can be used, depending on the indication. Radiofrequency (heating) or cryotherapy (freezing) probes can be used to cause a lesion in a nerve after precise localization with X-ray and nerve stimulation. Drugs with differing mechanisms of action, such as depot steroids, clonidine and opioids can be added to local anaesthetic. Historically, nerve block procedures were the cornerstone of pain clinic practice: their role has changed as more techniques for medical management are available and as pain relief is seen as part of a strategy of rehabilitation.

## Diagnostic nerve blocks

A diagnostic nerve block seeks evidence of pain relief following local anaesthetic block of a sensory nerve. The purpose of a diagnostic block is the identification of an anatomical lesion responsible for pain so that definitive treatment, such as surgery to a particular area or nerve destruction can be planned. Diagnostic blocks require precise localization of nerve to be of value. Inaccurate needle positioning gives a false indication of the likely pathology, and an overoptimistic interpretation of the results of definitive treatment. Even when a needle placement is satisfactory, there are several problems associated with the interpretation of diagnostic blocks, as follows:

- A placebo response.
- Needle placement is accurate but local anaesthetic has spread.
- The patient is responding to the systemic action of local anaesthetic.
- The nerve block includes the sympathetic nerve fibres and the block is not specific.

In an attempt to improve the accuracy of diagnostic block various recommendations have been made to overcome these problems. These are:

- Assessment is made by an observer who is unaware of the treatment.
- The duration of pain relief should be similar to the duration of action of the local anaesthetic.
- Pain relief that outlasts the anaesthetic duration may be due to other mechanisms not tested by the nerve block.
- The response to a specific sympathetic block should be ascertained first.
- Low volumes of local anaesthetic agent are used.
- The procedure is undertaken on more than one occasion.
- The patient understands the nature and purpose of the block.

Even when diagnostic nerve blocks are performed with attention to the above details, there can be further problems if it is assumed that nerve destruction or surgery will take away the pain:

- Pain relief can be obtained by nerve block in the area of referred pain rather than to the site of pain itself.
- Pain relief in practice may outlast the pharmacological action of local anaesthetic.
- The dorsal horn will respond to nerve destruction by becoming sensitized.
- A new pain is experienced.

Despite these limitations diagnostic nerve block of a somatic sensory nerve serves two other functions if a negative result is obtained:

- It may convince a patient of the futility of nerve destruction or surgery.
- It may indicate to the clinician that a central component to the pain exists.

It is also worth noting the comment of an authority on the subject who states that the practice of making a psychological assessment on the strength of a negative response to a diagnostic nerve block is 'an arrogance evolved from ignorance'.

## Therapeutic nerve blocks

Therapeutic nerve blocks include local anaesthetic, neurolytic and other drugs. *Local anaesthetic* on its own can break the 'vicious circle' of chronic pain. Once pain and spasm around a joint have been relieved, movement may become possible, and relief of disability and pain may outlast the pharmacological action of the anaesthetic. Such an action can be demonstrated after local anaesthetic block to nerves that provide sensory fibres to a joint, but whose motor fibres are not essential for movement of the joint. Examples include the use of obturator nerve block for the painful arthritic hip and suprascapular nerve block for the painful shoulder. The effect may be due to several factors:

- The initial movement around a joint stretches the surrounding structures leading to a return of normal range of movement. Limited movement due to pain may have led to a situation where capsular shrinkage and tendon shortening lead to pain on attempted movement.
- Constant nociceptive stimulation from the site of pain leads to secondary changes in the behaviour of the dorsal horn of the spinal cord, changes that may be reversed with block of the nociceptor afferents, even when this is only effective for a short period of time.
- The patient gains confidence in moving a limb that has been too painful to move.
- Block of the efferent sympathetic fibres may lead to a change in the behaviour of primary afferent nociceptors that are sensitive to the action of locally released noradrenaline. This effect may outlast the effect of afferent blockade.

Successful procedures may be repeated on an occasional basis. The anatomical explanation for referred pain is one of branching of primary afferents and converging of inputs onto a dorsal horn cell. It can be relieved by local anaesthetic to the site of referred pain. The success of this approach is due to block of tonically active nerve impulses which increase excitability of dorsal horn neurones. Some phenomena of referred pain are difficult to explain but may be treated by imaginative use of local anaesthetic. Examples include pain from angina referred to a recent thoracic vertebral fracture, and pain from sinusitis referred to recently filled teeth. Both visceral and musculoskeletal pains can be treated with therapeutic local anaesthetic nerve blocks of areas of referred pain. Visceral pathology may present with symptoms referred to the somatic dermatomes and local anaesthetic block here may be effective as pain relief.

## Nerve destruction techniques

Nerve lesions and neurolytic therapeutic injections of somatic sensory nerves should be performed only after a properly conducted diagnostic trial, as described above, unless clinical urgency (advanced malignancy) makes this approach inhumane or impractical. The major hazards of nerve destruction techniques are:

- Permanent motor block.
- Neuropathic pain as a consequence of dorsal horn sensitization.
- Accidental damage to structures adjacent to the target nerve.

*1.  Neurolytic substances*  in common use for peripheral block and autonomic ganglion block include phenol in aqueous solution and 50% alcohol. Phenol in glycerol is a hyperbaric preparation that can be used intrathecally and absolute alcohol is used as a hypobaric preparation intrathecally. The use of these depends upon the site of the required lesion relative to the site of injection. Thus phenol in glycerol is used to block the sacral nerve roots, the patient sitting with the injection performed in the lumbar region, whereas alcohol is used for lesions above the site of injection. Phenol has some local anaesthetic action, so is usually painless on injection, whereas alcohol causes intense pain. An aqueous solution of phenol can be used instead of alcohol.

*2.  Radiofrequency lesion generation*  is a technique by which high frequency electrical current (1 MHz or more) delivered via an insulated probe causes heating of adjacent tissue via an ionic effect, the current being dispersed via an earth electrode connected to the patient. The size of the resulting nerve lesion is affected by the dispersal of heat from the surrounding tissues, and, for normally vascularized tissue, is dependent upon the size of the electrode tip and the temperature measured at the tip. A temperature of 45°C is required to cause damage to C fibres. The resulting effect of heat dispersion through local blood flow is one of allowing precise temperature gradients around a probe of given size and tip temperature that is predictable and independent of the duration of current flow. Thus, for normally vascularized tissue, the radius of heat-induced damage to nociceptive fibres is precise and independent of the duration of current. For needles placed into intervertebral discs, the heat dissipation is much less rapid due to the avascularity of the disc, and the size of the lesion is dependent on the length of time for which current passes.

*3.  Pulsed radiofrequency*  is a new technique in which the current is delivered in pulses separated by intervals in which heat is dispersed. The result is the delivery of current, with ionic effects, but with the temperature of the tissue around the needle tip kept at about 43°C. Reports of long-acting pain relief, presumably consequent on C fibre inactivation have been claimed. The mechanism by which pulsed radiofrequency current delivers a nerve lesion effect is uncertain: heat inactivation or heat-mediated destruction of the nociceptor fibres is clearly not involved. It is thought that such techniques may be particularly valuable for producing nerve lesions in target tissue where nociceptor fibres and somatosensory fibres subserving touch exist in close proximity and where there may be hazards of causing a heat lesion of the latter. Thus pulsed radiofrequency techniques have been claimed to be of value in dorsal root ganglion denervation procedures and in peripheral neuromata.

## Related topics of interest

Back pain – injections (p. 35); Therapy – nerve blocks: autonomic (p. 176).

# THERAPY – NEUROSURGICAL TECHNIQUES

*Paul Eldridge*

This chapter is not intended as a comprehensive account of all the neurosurgical procedures for pain; rather it is intended to explain the rationale of neurosurgery for pain, and illustrate some of its potential. One of the most important roles of a neurosurgeon involved in surgery for pain is to be certain that surgically remediable pathology has not been missed – in the case of 'chronic' sciatica this may be a simple lumbar disc prolapse – more rarely 'trigeminal neuralgia' may represent the facial pain from an acoustic or even trigeminal schwannoma. As far as specialist pain clinic practice is concerned, procedures may involve quite specialized techniques drawn from different areas of neurosurgery such as spinal neurosurgery or stereotactic and image-guided techniques. The 'pain' neurosurgeon thus requires considerable general and specialist expertise. A fully equipped neurosurgical facility is of course required, with facilities for intraoperative neurophysiological monitoring.

Neurosurgery for the relief of persistent pain began in the 19th century with root sections and later cordotomy. Pain relief was dominated by these methods until the second half of the 20th century when advances in analgesics, including anticonvulsants, psychotropics and specific opiate preparations, were associated with the rapid development of pain clinics and hospices. There was then a virtual cessation in the practice of neurosurgery for pain relief.

In the last 20 years the development of more precise, safe, effective and low-morbidity techniques has resulted in a renewed interest in neurosurgery for the relief of pain when medication has proved inadequate or intolerable. These advances include percutaneous techniques and non-destructive/augmentative techniques such as electrical stimulation or the implantation of sophisticated devices for drug delivery. The percutaneous techniques were particularly suited to an anaesthetic training, from which specialty many pain practitioners came.

The procedures performed are of four types:

> *1. Correct structural problem.* Microvascular decompression (MVD) for trigeminal neuralgia (TGN), spinal fusions for instability, discectomy, tumour resections – these procedures are discussed elsewhere in the book.
>
> *2. Non-destructive or augmentative such as electrical stimulation.* At many sites in the nervous system, though most commonly the spinal cord; at its most sophisticated this includes stimulation of deep brain structures, as discussed elsewhere in the book.
>
> *3. Destructive procedures.* Radio-frequency lesioning, root sections, open cordotomy, commisurotomy, DREZ, medullary tractotomy, thalamotomy and pituitary ablation; some of these are discussed below.
>
> *4. Implantation of intrathecal infusion devices.* The use of intrathecal baclofen for multiple sclerosis and opioids for cancer depends on a surgically implanted device.

In the first category, apart from MVD (see below), the examples may appear at first sight unrelated to the specialty of pain. However most spinal neurosurgeons regard lumbar micro-discetomy as simply a procedure for pain relief.

The distinction between destructive and non-destructive procedures is important since destructive procedures are most appropriate for treatment of persistent pain due to malignancy, where life expectancy is limited and are little used for non-malignant pains. The reason for this is that relapse rates are high after destructive procedures; there is a risk of neurological deficit and therefore disability; and new syndromes (particularly dysaesthetic-type pains) may arise after destruction of the nervous system at either peripheral or central levels, though more particularly after peripheral lesions.

Another underlying and related philosophy is that low-risk procedures are to be attempted before high-risk procedures even if the success rate of the former is poor; thus deep brain lesions or stimulation tend to be last resort options. Finally, it is important that a multidisciplinary approach occurs: in the author's unit this is achieved by joint ward rounds and clinics between anaesthetic, neurological and neurosurgical pain specialists, and involving nurse specialists, and the pain management team.

## Lesions

It has been mentioned above that lesions for pain are to be avoided because of the risk of pain recurrence; development of late dysaesthetic pains and of course the inevitable loss of function that may occur. An example of this is lesioning the lateral cutaneous nerve of the thigh for meralgia paraesthetica. Although widely practised, the outcomes of this are poor and include all three of the complications mentioned above. One exception is perhaps partial sensory rhizotomy performed for trigeminal neuralgia; here although there is loss of function there is good pain relief which is maintained in a high percentage of cases, though not all. Some lesion techniques are now discussed in greater detail.

## Dorsal root entry zone (DREZ)

There are a number of destructive lesions of the spinal cord designed to alleviate pain. Procedures such as cordotomy and commissural myelotomy of these are reserved for cases of cancer. The DREZ lesion is unusual in that it is used for chronic pain due to non-malignant causes. Cordotomy and commissural myelotomy certainly have relapse rates, and like DREZ carry risk of significant physical disability. Although cervical cordotomy can be performed percutaneously in the neck, elsewhere an open laminectomy is needed.

## DREZ lesion

### Historical

It was first introduced by Sindou in 1972 as a treatment for neuropathic pain and spasticity. He coined the term microsurgical selective posterior rhizotomy. The lesion was also popularized by Nashold in 1976 who used radiofrequency technology to create the lesion in the dorsal root entry zone – hence the acronym 'DREZ' particularly for brachial plexus lesions.

## Syndromes

The best indications seem to be brachial plexus avulsion injuries; well localized cancer pain as in Pancoast syndrome (carcinoma of the lung apex associated with brachial neuralgia), cauda equina and spinal cord lesions for pain corresponding to segmental lesions, peripheral nerve lesions, amputations and herpes zoster provided the predominant component of the pain is paroxysmal and associated with allodynia. It can also be used for spasticity, and for hyperactive neuropathic bladder.

## Operation

This is an open neurosurgical procedure requiring a laminectomy with opening of the dura to expose the spinal cord. The DREZ region is identified from the position of the dorsal rootlets; the target for the lesion is immediately anterior to this point. A lesion of depth 2–3 mm is created affecting Rexed layers I–IV. This may be difficult to identify when the roots have been avulsed as is the case in brachial plexus injuries. There may also be problems in identifying the correct level and intraoperative fluoroscopy can be used. Some employ intraoperative neurophysiological monitoring of somatosensory evoked potentials in order to guard against unintentional damage to the dorsal columns.

## Risks

The main complication is ipsilateral leg weakness, though there may also be ipsilateral loss of sensation. Some subjective loss of sensation and/or weakness may occur in as many as 60% of cases and be significant in up to 10%. Loss of bladder control can occur albeit rarely. For these reasons DREZ lesion is often only attempted as a last resort; it may follow attempts at spinal cord stimulation even if this is not thought likely to succeed.

## Outcomes

For brachial plexus lesions success rates of 70% are reported with long-term follow-up of between 1–8 years. Rates of 50–70% are found for other indications; where relief is obtained it does seem to be maintained. However, the experience in the author's unit is for a tendency to relapse with time, a finding in keeping with most other ablative or destructive techniques for the treatment of pain.

Results for post-herpetic neuralgia are much less encouraging; although initial success rates of about 60% are observed this falls to only 25% with longer follow-up.

# Cordotomy

## Indications

This procedure is performed almost exclusively for malignant pain. The ideal candidate has pain around the torso or into the lower limbs on one side. Bilateral cases can be considered, but significant side-effects then accepted.

## Methods

It can be performed either percutaneously or at open operation. The aim is to cut the anterior spinothalamic tract.

The percutaneous method is performed by lateral cervical puncture between C1 and C2; an approach originally used for cervical myelograms. The procedure is performed under fluoroscopic control. Contrast is injected which enables the ligamentum denticulatum to be identified so that a radiofrequency needle can be inserted. Stimulation is carried out to confirm hypoalgesia in the desired area (the patient typically experiences a feeling of warmth rather than parasthesiae) and then a lesion can be made.

The open method requires a general anaesthetic and a laminectomy above the level of the pain. The spinal cord is exposed; rotated gently using the ligamentum denticulatum and an incision made in the contralateral anterior quadrant to the pain. The depth of the lesion is approximately 2–3 mm, judged by the operator. The procedure is quite simple and of much lower morbidity than the description might suggest, though not competitive to the percutaneous method.

Complications of both methods are ipsilateral muscle weakness. If performed bilaterally, then loss of bladder function should be included. Risk to respiration, particularly if performed at the cervical level is significant. If performed for chest pain for lung carcinoma, then the respiratory function on the side of the pain may already be compromised. Therefore the production of weakness on the 'good' side may be significant. If bilateral cervical lesions are performed then the patient's respiratory centres can be affected so that 'Ondine's curse' may develop – here respiration only occurs whilst the patient is awake. This leads to an indication for open, high-thoracic cordotomy when a previous contralateral percutaneous cervical cordotomy has been performed. How high this cordotomy should be must be judged; lower in order to preserve function, but as the fibres may cross over as much as eight levels, too low will result in loss of efficacy.

## Results

It is a highly effective, and probably underused method of pain control in patients with advanced carcinoma. It should be accepted that pain relief will last for only a few months. In the context of patients with advanced carcinoma this is acceptable. In addition the patient may already be disabled by the disease so that side-effects are also acceptable. Although the procedure has been performed historically for non-cancer pain this cannot be recommended.

## Commissural myelotomy

The spinal cord is divided thereby cutting the pain fibres as they cross over. The indication is for pelvic pain from advanced carcinoma; it is rarely performed as a bilateral cordotomy would achieve the same goal in the rare circumstance of failure of medical management. The morbidity is quite high with effectively loss of use of the lower limbs, and bladder and bowel control.

# Intrathecal drug delivery systems

There is increasing use of such systems.

## Indications

These may be divided into two and it is convenient to consider them separately.

*1. Baclofen for the management of spasticity.* The indication is provoked by pain from the continuing muscle spasm; additional benefits are improvement in function and for disabled bed-bound patients ease of nursing care. The aetiology of the spasm is often multiple sclerosis, but occasionally it is used for non-progressive conditions such as the aftermath of a spinal cord injury; cervical or thoracic stenosis or prolapsed cervical or thoracic disc; after thoracic cord lesions such as a disc, or tumour. Since cervical myelopathy tends to occur in an elderly population it rarely provides an indication for pump implantation.

*2. Opioids, or opioids in combination with a number of drugs including local anaesthetics, clonidine and NMDA antagonists such as ketamine.* These are used for malignant pain, and more recently it is being increasingly used for non-malignant pain. The former use is straightforward, and the indication is where other routes of administration for the control of pain are ineffective. The use for non-malignant pain is much more controversial though success is obtained.

## Methods

A catheter is placed intrathecally and connected to a pump placed usually in the anterior abdominal wall. These pumps are now quite sophisticated and can be programmed to deliver different dose rates, varying these across a 24-hour period and to deliver bolus doses. Making use of this facility does require the services of an appropriate infrastructure – pain specialist nurses able to program the pump and the reader will be aware of regulatory issues surrounding the safe administration of intrathecal drugs. Non-programmable pumps are also available, but the only advantage of these is their lower cost. The dose rate can only be altered by refilling the pump with a different concentration of drug. Regular follow-up by the implanting surgeon is required as loss of efficacy may be due to a problem with the pump; the commonest one being breakage or detachment of the catheter from the pump. With a pump in situ near normal activities of daily life are possible.

Pumps must be refilled at approximately 3 month intervals; it does not seem practical to extend this time period owing to the stability of the different drugs at body temperature. For patients with malignant disease, with poor life expectancy, an intrathecal or epidural catheter connected to an external pump is acceptable.

For both pain and spasticity trial doses are used to confirm that the patient responds and to allow patient and carers to see what benefits may be achieved.

## Results – spasticity

The results are excellent. The dose must be titrated to allow a balance between function and relief of spasticity. Often the programming facility is used to increase the dose at night when spasms are a problem but decrease in the day when more muscle tone is needed for transfers etc.

**Results – pain**

No controlled trials exist, though observational studies find good results. An evidence-based review exists (see Further reading). Results are excellent for cancer pain, but much more controversial for non-cancer pain. A comprehensive evaluation is required before considering patients for non-maligant pain, particularly if chronic opioid usage is involved. This will include in addition to trial of the method, psychological assessments.

## Further reading

Polyanalgesic Consensus Conference 2000. *Journal of Pain and Symptom Management*, 2000; **20**(2): S1–50.

White JC, Sweet WH. *Pain and the neurosurgeon.* Charles C. Thomas, Springfield, Illinois, 1969.

## Related topics of interest

Cancer – nerve blocks (p. 53); Neuralgia – trigeminal and glossopharyngeal (p. 107).

# THERAPY – OPIOIDS IN CHRONIC PAIN

*Andrew Severn, Barrie Tait*

The use of opioids in pain of non-malignant origin is controversial and depends on a proper understanding of the nature of chronic pain, and the strategy of its management. Patients with chronic pain who take opioids must understand the rationale for the use and be prepared to be an active partner in the management of the condition.

Opioid drugs are analgesics, the action of which is mediated via receptors in the central nervous system. Three types of receptors are involved in the analgesia of opioids: these are the $\mu$, $\kappa$ and $\delta$ receptors. Receptors are identified in the brain, the spinal cord, and afferent neurones. Receptor sensitivity may be enhanced by an inflammatory process and reduced by neuropathic pain mechanisms. Some of the action of opioid drugs may be mediated indirectly via an action on adrenergic and serotoninergic modulation of the spinal cord. Presynaptic action on the primary afferent C fibre is believed to be an important site of action. Morphine, local anaesthetic, ketamine and NSAIDs may have synergistic actions in preventing the process of neuronal sensitization.

All clinically useful opioids are $\mu$ agonists, but use has been made of partial agonists such as buprenorphine and nalbuphine. Buprenorphine is a partial $\mu$ agonist, and nalbuphine a partial $\kappa$ agonist which has antagonistic actions at the $\mu$ receptor. Tramadol is a $\mu$, $\kappa$ and $\delta$ agonist which stimulates the release of serotonin and inhibits the reuptake of noradrenaline. It is useful to consider opioids as weak or strong depending on their relative efficacy. Codeine is a weak opioid, whose effects are maximum at about 200 mg per day. Strong opioids include morphine, its prodrug diamorphine, methadone, fentanyl, oxycodone and hydromorphone. Fentanyl is available as a transdermal patch, providing 72 h of continuous delivery.

## Side-effects

The effects of opioids when used for acute control of the nociceptive pain of injury are well known and include respiratory depression, sedation, nausea and pupillary constriction. However in the context of the chronic pain sufferer these physiological events are of less importance (and need not be considered) than the issues of dependency, tolerance, and addiction which are considered here. There is ample observational work on large cohort studies to show that the extensive use of opioids for the control of acute pain, for example in war casualties, does not lead to dependency in the longer term.

*1. Dependence* has been described in volunteers who do not have pain, and in subjects who have a history of addiction to opioids as a consequence of recreational use. Dependence is, however, poorly understood in chronic pain sufferers. The consequences of withdrawing opioids from patients who have become accustomed to high doses after, for example, a cure of a painful condition or a nerve block to relieve the pain are said to be different from those of withholding opioids from subjects who have taken recreational opioids. Although physiological changes are to be expected and include gastrointestinal disturbance and chills, they do not have the same psychological consequences for the patient as the devastating symptoms associated with drug withdrawal in the habitual drug user, and they are not said to be associated with a craving for drug and drug-seeking behaviour. The claims that certain opioids are to be preferred because of the lack of dependency potential have to be judged against these observations. Although different drugs, and different routes of administration may result in variations of plasma drug level and CNS effects, the concept that any one opioid drug has an inherent greater or lesser danger of provoking dependency is not supported by available evidence. Rather it is the route of administration and the effect of variations of drug concentrations and effect that may be responsible for a tendency to dependency, and with it, the risk of addiction. Such a mechanism may be mediated by the dopamine pathways of the mesolimbic system and the periaqueductal grey cells. Rapidly rising drug levels in this part of the brain lead to an increase in dopaminergic activity that may promote behaviour to repeat the experience.

2. **Tolerance** is the diminution of effect of drug with time, or the need to increase dose to maintain an effect. Tolerance is considered as a normal and expected response and not of harmful significance. In observing the opioid requirement of the patient with a static disease process, tolerance results in the progressive reduction of effect and the need for an increased dose. It is said that there is a ceiling for tolerance and that, once this is reached, further demands for increase have to be explained in other ways, such as worsening pathology, psychological distress or depression or the unmasking of a tendency to addiction. Tolerance extends the usefulness of the drug, since tolerance to side-effects also occurs. Tolerance is a result of several mechanisms, of which the following are notable:

- A pharmocokinetic action, such as the induction of enzymes, or the accumulation of metabolites with antagonist properties (e.g. morphine-3-glucuronide).
- A pharmacodynamic action that results from changes in the drug receptor.

3. **Addiction** is a term reserved for the behaviour associated with the compulsive use of drugs, without regard for the clinical indication, and despite harm. It can conveniently be considered a brain disease, involving neurological mechanisms in the 'pleasure pathway' of the medial forebrain bundle and associated structures, and with dopamine as the main neurotransmitter. Various theories of 'nature vs nurture' have been propounded to explain and/or excuse patterns in behaviour of groups at risk of addiction. It seems clear that both factors, and the nature of the substance for which the addict craves, determine the development of addictive behaviour. Thus alcohol may be considered a drug for which the genetic predisposition to addictive behaviour is important, the drug itself being less so, but cocaine has a high inherent addictive potential and genetic makeup does not protect the casual user from a serious risk of addiction.

The extent to which the opioid drugs used in clinical practice have the potential for unmasking addictive behaviour is unclear. There are many observational studies that support the idea of patients maintained on long-term opioids for considerable lengths of time without evidence of addictive behaviour. It should be remembered however, that there exist in society a proportion of patients who have at some time abused drugs and whose behaviour with treatment will need careful monitoring. There is also the real threat posed to patients who have supplies of opioid drugs in their homes or on their person from criminal elements.

Thus the management of chronic pain of non-malignant origin with opioids remains controversial, not least because of the ethical difficulties involved in conducting proper randomized controlled trials in opioid naïve patients with chronic pain. The use of drugs with a 'low ceiling' effect, such as codeine or a partial agonist, may protect the prescriber against fears of 'feeding a drug habit', but may not be the most appropriate for the patient or the condition. The claim that tramadol has a good record in respect of addictive behaviour is based on observations of opioid preferences in addicts and is probably inappropriate to apply to the chronic pain population, for reasons given above. Far better that a decision be made that the pain is likely or not likely to respond to opioids, that other issues in respect of distress or illness behaviour dealt with and a decision made early to use or not to use this class of drugs than to rely on a theoretical ceiling effect to avoid the complications of dependency. The route and timing of administration is important. Avoidance of high peak drug levels in the brain mandates the use of slow-release preparations administered by the oral or transdermal route, rather than 'as required' doses by the intramuscular or buccal route. Similarly, it is important to recognize that if there is a need for a strong opioid, there is a continuing requirement. The use of these drugs presupposes an incurable nociceptive cause and a brain whose receptors will have become used to the presence of drug. There is little logic in the occasional use of opioid for chronically painful conditions, unless the natural history of the underlying condition is characterized by fluctuations in nociceptive stimulus, as in for example the patient with recurrent urinary tract stone formation or sickle cell disease.

Given that it may be appropriate for patients with chronic pain and a normal life expectancy to receive opioids, it is worth considering how the process is monitored. A careful lookout has to be made for behaviour that is suspicious of wrong usage. The term pseudoaddiction is used to describe the behaviour of the pain sufferer who achieves some, but suboptimal, pain relief from opioids and requests more. Requests for increases in dose may be plausible or less so: the way in which these requests are phrased may indicate whether or not the patient is appropriately using the drug. A preference for one particular type or brand of opioid analgesic may be justifiable, as may be the practice of hoarding of the drug to use when the pain is severe. However, bizarre explanations of the fate of drugs which were prescribed but never used: 'the dog ate it', 'I left it on the train' should raise suspicions of wrong usage.

The acceptability and availability of opioids varies greatly between countries and reflects the importance that fear of wrong use is held in society. This fear may be sanctioned by the state, whose doctors may be viewed with suspicion if they prescribe opioids. Other societal beliefs about the dangers of opioids may influence the acceptability of the drugs. A sample poll of the British public in the wake of a sensational conviction of a doctor who used morphine for multiple murder demonstrated a fear of being prescribed morphine. Conversely, the availability of alternative opioids such as fentanyl and oxycodone that are not recognized as morphine-like substances by the public may lead to preference for one particular opioid that is little to do with the quality of pain relief afforded by the drug. In this respect it is difficult to interpret the findings of a recent randomized, but necessarily unblinded, crossover trial comparing slow-release oral morphine with transdermal fentanyl in which a 'preference' for transdermal fentanyl was expressed.

Some organizations and countries have proposed guidelines for the prescription of opioids for pain of non-malignant origin. In general terms these guidelines follow the principles outlined above: that opioids may be useful, that other methods of tackling the pain should be considered, that the pain should be nociceptive, that coexisting psychological morbidity should be treated, and that a careful watch should be kept for the appearance of symptoms of dependency or the behaviour of abuse. Some guidelines recommend two independent doctors sanctioning the prescription, and a contract with the patient. Whatever the guidelines, it is important that the patient is a full partner in discussion, knows that the drug is being used to modify, rather than cure the pain, and agrees to be monitored.

## Further reading

Allan L, Hays H, Jensen N-H *et al.* Randomised crossover trial of transdermal fentanyl and sustained release oral morphine for treating chronic non-cancer pain. *British Medical Journal*, 2001; **322:** 1154–8.

Hymes JA. Chemical dependency issues in patients with low back pain. *Seminars in Spine Surgery.* WB Saunders 1996; **8**(3): 202–7.

Portenoy RK. Opioid tolerance and responsiveness: research findings and clinical observations. In: Gebbart GF, Hammond DL, Jensen TS (eds). *Proceedings of the 7th World Congress on Pain, Progress in Pain Research and Management, Vol. 2.* Seattle: IASP Press, 1994; pp. 595–620.

## Related topic of interest

Cancer – opioid drugs (p. 56).

# THERAPY – PHYSICAL

*Barrie Tait*

Physical therapies are widely used in the management of chronic pain, particularly a pain of musculoskeletal origin. Physical therapies can be primarily directed to modulation of the pain control system, such as with acupuncture. Or they can be primarily directed to movement of the pain-sensitive structures, either in a general manner, such as with exercise, or more specifically, as with manual treatments of mobilization and manipulation. Rest, either general, such as bed rest or local rest, such as with the case of lumbar supports, can be considered as physical therapies. There have been randomized controlled studies of these therapies but their quality has tended to be poor and so systematic reviews have provided only limited support for their use.

## Bed rest and lumbar supports

Since the publication in 1863 of John Hilton's *Rest and Pain* there has been an emphasis on rest as a key modality in the management of pain, especially pain of musculoskeletal origin. Systematic reviews of randomized controlled studies of bed rest for acute low back pain with the outcome measures of pain, functional status, recovery and return to work have shown that bed rest, compared with advice to stay active, at best has small positive effects and at worst might have small negative effects on acute low back pain. Lumbar supports are used in the treatment of low back pain patients to make the impairment and disability vanish or decrease. However the systematic review of therapeutic trials showed that there is limited evidence that lumbar supports are more effective than no treatment, and it was unclear if lumbar supports are more effective than other interventions for treatment of low back pain.

## Exercise therapy

Exercises as therapy can be used as a sole therapy or part of a more complex programme, such as Back Schools, or cognitive behavioural interdisciplinary programmes. Systematic review of studies using pain intensity, functional states, overall improvement and return to work as outcomes measures did not indicate that specific exercises are effective for the treatment of acute low back pain. Exercises may be helpful for chronic low back pain patients to increase return to normal daily activities and work.

## Physiotherapy

There are many techniques and procedures for manual therapy for pain of musculoskeletal origin, particularly spinal pain. The two standard approaches are mobilization and manipulation. Mobilization involves the systematic application of force of progressively increasing magnitude, ostensibly to a selected joint or spinal motion segment. Manipulation involves the sudden application of a single, forceful thrust to a selected joint or spinal motion segment. There have been a number of systematic reviews of these treatments. A recent review concluded that there is limited evidence that manipulation is more effective than a placebo treatment.

In the evaluation of physiotherapy for the management of chronic pain the lack of evidence of efficacy does not imply that physiotherapy has been shown to be ineffective. It does suggest that as a sole modality physiotherapy is very limited. However, as a key component of a structured cognitive behavioural programme, the positive systematic reviews of this type of treatment would strongly support the use of physiotherapy modalities in the broader psychosocial approach.

## Acupuncture and massage

The modulation of the pain control system may be achieved by a range of peripheral stimulation techniques. Two of the most commonly used are acupuncture and massage. Systematic reviews do not indicate that acupuncture is effective for the treatment of back pain. Other systematic reviews have concluded that the efficacy of acupuncture in the treatment of chronic pain remains doubtful.

The quality of controlled trials of massage have not been high enough to definitively evaluate its effect. A systematic review concluded that there is insufficient evidence to recommend massage as a stand-alone treatment for non-specific low back pain.

The collective results of the systematic reviews of physical therapy can be interpreted that their widespread use must be explained by other factors than simply their physical effects.

# Further reading

Nachenson A, Jonsson E (eds). *Neck and Back Pain: The Scientific Evidence of Causes, Diagnosis and Treatment*. Philadelphia; Lippincott Williams and Wilkins; 2000.

# Systematic reviews

Furlan AD, Brosseau L, Welch V, Wong J. *Massage for low back pain (Cochrane Review)*. In: The Cochrane Library, Issue 4, 2000.

Gross AR, Aker PD, Goldsmith CH, Pelosis P. *Physical medicine modalities for mechanical neck disorders (Cochrane Review)*. In: The Cochrane Library, Issue 4, 2000.

Hagen KB, Hilde G, Jamtveldt G, Winnem M. *Bed rest for acute low pain and sciatica (Cochrane Review)*. In: The Cochrane Library, Issue 4, 2000.

van Tulder MW, Jellema P, van Popper MNM, Nachenson AL, Fouter LM. *Lumbar supports for presentation and treatment of low back pain (Cochrane Review)*. In: The Cochrane Library, Issue 4, 2000.

van Tulder MW, van Malmivara A, Esmail R, Koes BW. *Exercise therapy for low back pain (Cochrane Review)*. In: The Cochrane Library, Issue 4, 2000.

van Tulder MW, van Cherkin DC, Berman B, Lao L, Koes BW. *Acupuncture for low back pain (Cochrane Review)*. In: The Cochrane Library, Issue 4, 2000.

van Tulder MW, Kees BW, Bouter M. Conservative treatment of acute and chronic non-specific low back pain. A systematic review of randomised controlled trials of the most common interventions. *Spine*, 1997; **22**: 2128–56.

# THERAPY – PSYCHOLOGICAL

*Andrew Severn*

The aim of psychological management is one of changing the perception of sufferers, so that rather than considering themselves to be suffering from chronic illness, they consider themselves to be well and coping, and responsible for the maintenance of their own health.

The psychological management of pain addresses those features of the chronic pain syndrome described as cognitive and behavioural features. It does not attempt to provide relief from pain, although relief of pain is sometimes recorded as a result of treatment. Psychological management is sometimes deferred until all possible medical treatments have been concluded. This approach has the advantage that the sufferer cannot approach psychological treatments with an ambivalent attitude and has to accept that there is no medical cure for the pain. However, this particular approach has two problems. Firstly, successive attempts to treat pain symptoms without addressing the psychosocial dimension risks making the distress worse with every failed intervention. Secondly, the approach engenders in the minds of all involved an unnecessary distinction, a dualism, between the medical cause and the psychosocial presentation. It has been suggested that psychosocial features are of relevance to the outcome of painful conditions within a short time of initial presentation (in the presentation of back pain these factors are referred to as 'yellow flags'), and that early intervention might prevent progression to a chronic pain syndrome.

Interview and self-rating questionnaires may describe the sufferer in terms of affective, cognitive, behavioural or functional impairment. Individualized treatment plans can be designed. An efficient use of resources is a Pain Management Programme which provides psychological management within a group setting. An advantage of this approach is the peer pressure that can be applied on members of the group. Programmes are typically outpatient activities, but inpatient programmes are suitable for isolated areas or where the patients are most disabled. The precise subject matter of programmes varies with the skill-mix and interest of the staff, but in general terms the treatment is termed cognitive behavioural therapy. An outline of the treatment of cognitive behavioural therapy is as follows, and is 'taught' or 'practiced' within the context of a course of group instruction over a period of weeks or months.

## Information

An explanation of the nature of chronic pain is necessary to overcome fears that pain is a sign of harm that requires rest. The concept of chronic pain as a disease as distinct from a symptom is difficult to grasp. Inadequate explanations or the unguarded use of medical jargon may have resulted in false beliefs about the presence of progressive disease. Inadequate understanding of the nature and purpose of investigations and treatment lead the pain sufferer to expect further tests or surgery. It is helpful to have an explanation from an expert about the limitations of medical treatment. Explanations about the role of analgesics, in particular about the hazards of using a 'pain contingent' or 'as required' dosing strategy, are also useful.

## Coping skills

Strategies for dealing with exacerbations of pain can be introduced. The gate control theory of pain modulation can be used as a model to explain that many factors influence the perception of pain. Distraction techniques encourage the use of intensive mental or pleasurable activity, including relaxation techniques, to overcome the pain experience. Distraction techniques encourage the patient to develop an 'internal' way of managing distress, rather than relying on 'external' factors, such as analgesics or the physical attentions of a partner or health professional.

## Mood modification

The effect of mood on the pain experience can be addressed by encouraging patients to challenge negative thoughts which accompany disability or an exacerbation of pain.

## Activity modification

Inappropriate expectations of ability and fear of activity are features of the pain experience that need specific attention. The two concepts introduced are goal setting and pacing. Goal setting refers to a target for physical activity that is agreed between patient and professional, and pacing is the tactic by which this target is achieved. In the case of the patient who undertakes excess activity when pain is controlled and is then disabled by pain as a consequence of this activity, paced activity demands a disciplined approach to rest breaks and exercise. Activity goals during a programme are agreed by mutual consent: the patient is encouraged to start activity at a level compatible with pre-existing fitness and to increase this level progressively.

## Behaviour modification

The psychological management of pain addresses those behaviours that cause the sufferer to become dependent on others. The overprotective partner is encouraged to allow the pain sufferer to undertake activities, and needs education about all the issues outlined above. Pain behaviour can be a threat to normal social functioning. It can be reduced by responses which pay little attention to the behaviour. This approach sees pain behaviours as responses that have been reinforced by inappropriate attention, such as encouragement to rest, continued investigation to find non-existent pathology, and continued attempts to cure the pain.

## Outcomes of cognitive behavioural therapy

Notwithstanding the difficulty in designing appropriate clinical trials comparing cognitive behavioural therapy with 'standard' treatment, there seems to be good evidence for efficacy in a number of different chronic pain conditions. A recent systematic review has reviewed 25 controlled trials. In these trials control groups remained on waiting lists or received basic medical, family or physiotherapy support. It is possible that many such control patients concomitantly received therapy from other therapists not included in the trial teams. The review examined outcomes studied by the trials in the reporting of pain experience, mood, coping strategies, activity levels, and overt pain behaviour. In addition some trials examined the impact of cognitive behavioural therapy on fitness, social role functioning and use of healthcare system, including drug use. The review concluded that outcomes in many of these criteria were improved where cognitive behavioural therapy was included. In practical terms there is evidence to support cognitive behavioural therapy for conditions including low back pain, irritable bowel syndrome and conditions in which pain may be associated, such as the chronic fatigue syndrome.

## Systematic reviews

Evans G, Richards S. *Low back pain: an evaluation of therapeutic interventions.* University of Bristol, Health Care Evaluation Unit, 1996; 176.

Morley S, Eccleston C, Williams A. Systematic review and meta-analysis of randomised controlled trials of cognitive behaviour therapy and behaviour therapy for chronic pain in adults, excluding headache. *Pain,* 1999; **80:** 1–13.

## Related topics of interest

Assessment of chronic pain – psychosocial (p. 25); Back pain – medical management (p. 29); Gastrointestinal pain (p. 80); Musculoskeletal pain syndromes (p. 95).

# THERAPY – SPINAL-CORD AND BRAIN STIMULATION

*Paul Eldridge*

The recent use of electrical stimulation to relieve pain dates back to 1967, when spinal cord stimulation was first attempted by Shealy and co-workers, the logic for this following on from Melzack and Wall's gate control theory for pain published in 1965.

## Methods and sites

The commonest site for stimulation is the spinal cord. Stimulation can also be delivered to sites within the brain (such as the thalamus) or occasionally over the motor cortex of the brain. Stimulation can be used for control of conditions other than pain such as, spasticity, bladder control in multiple sclerosis (MS), peripheral vascular disease (PVD) and angina. In addition to benefits of reducing some of the symptoms of the disease, these techniques may also provide pain relief.

TNS (transcutaneous stimulation) is considered elsewhere in another chapter in this book. As a form of spinal cord stimulation it is less invasive than the techniques considered here.

## Spinal cord

### Physiology

The mechanism of spinal cord stimulation is unknown. Three possible mechanisms have been suggested. Stimulation using currents, voltages and frequencies typically in use is shown to activate the dorsal column fibres. Larger fibres are preferentially activated, though the spinal sympathetic pathways are also activated.

- In the first of these mechanisms it is suggested that antidromic activation of dorsal column fibres 'closes the gate'. This was the original logic behind the development of the use of SCS.
- The second mechanism involves supraspinal pathways. Stimulation passes up the dorsal columns to the anterior pre-tectal nuclei in the brain stem, and is relayed back down to the spinal cord via the dorsal longitudinal funiculus, where the pain pathways are modulated.
- Lastly, spinal cord stimulation acts by stimulating adrenergic sympathetic neurones. This probably accounts for the effects on blood flow seen in peripheral vascular disease and angina, and on bladder function seen in multiple sclerosis.

However none of these mechanisms has been proven, and all may be important. The effects on blood flow seem separate from the effects on pain. The dorsal columns are important as pain relief is not obtained unless paraesthesiae are produced in the affected area; indeed the precise position of the electrode is crucial to success of the technique. The observation that paraesthesiae must be perceived by the patient argues for a supra-spinal mechanism. Some studies have been made of neurochemical changes resulting from SCS; most of these are inconsistent, though rises in noradrenaline, substance P and 5HT have been observed. In contrast to TNS, the action of SCS is unaffected by naloxone.

## Methods

An electrode array is positioned over the midline of the spinal cord in the epidural space. The usual minimum surface area of the electrodes is about 6–8 mm². At least two electrodes of opposite polarity are required, but it is more usual to use an array of four or more electrodes. The current trend is to use an increasing number of electrodes. There must be at least one electrode of each polarity but thereafter any combination of polarity, and number of electrodes in use is possible. The electrodes are activated in one of two ways. The more usual practice is to connect the electrodes to a battery-powered internal transmitter. The alternative is to use a receiver implanted subcutaneously (usually the flank). This receiver is powered by induction from an external transmitter, using an aerial attached to a battery-powered transmitter. However these systems are becoming less and less used. The fully internal systems do not require the patient to continuously have a receiver taped to the body; this allows much more freedom of activity – especially when sleeping, or in daily activities. The disadvantage is that the battery must be renewed periodically – usually about every 3–5 years depending on use.

The system can be programmed in detail; programmable parameters include varying frequency of stimulus, amplitude, duration of stimulus pulse and which electrode in the array is active and its polarity.

## Surgical procedure

Electrodes can be implanted percutaneously, or at open operation. Whatever the method, positioning of the electrode is crucial. Paraesthesiae must be elicited in the area of the pain, and there should not be over-stimulation of areas unaffected by pain as such stimulation can prove unpleasant. As frequency, pulse width and amplitude of stimulus increase so does the area covered.

## Percutaneous method

Percutaneously the electrode is passed down a Tuohy needle into the epidural space. Current designs mean this electrode must be cylindrical so that the electrode contacts run in a line. Once the electrode is in position, the remainder of the system can be implanted making a subcutaneous tunnel from the back round to the flank where the receiver is usually positioned. The whole procedure can be carried out under local anaesthetic. The advantage of this system is that it is less invasive, and because it is carried out under local anaesthetic the correct position of the electrode can be confirmed by stimulation during the procedure. The major disadvantage is that it is difficult to keep such electrodes in a constant position, and this is particularly true in the neck. Movement may then result in sudden and unpredictable decreases or increases in stimulation; the latter are extremely unpleasant for the patient. The method is used when the patient is unfit for general anaesthesia (e.g. SCS for angina), or when expertise necessary to carry out surgical implantation is unavailable.

## Surgical implantation

An open operation under general anaesthesia, and partial laminectomy is required when surgical electrodes are to be implanted. Position is held much better, and because a larger electrode surface is available the system provides better and more controllable stimulation. Accurate positioning of the electrode relies upon information from a pre-operative trial, or from placing an electrode with a large enough array so that a given combination of electrodes will stimulate the desired area. If electrodes are placed in a partly transverse direction, then two or more electrodes can be programmed from the four available in most arrays to stimulate the desired area.

## Trial procedures

Because a major procedure may be involved, and because the stimulator equipment is quite costly, many practitioners will undertake a trial of stimulation prior to permanent implantation. An electrode is passed into the epidural space under local anaesthesia using a Tuohy needle and brought out through the skin to an external power source. The position of the electrode can be adjusted at stimulation and also by staged withdrawal in the ward. The trial normally lasts 5–7 days, but can under certain circumstances last several weeks. It may be necessary to send the patient home to ensure an accurate trial; this may be particularly important in Raynaud's disease as the subject may need to experience a cold environment to provoke the symptoms!

The case against a trial procedure is that it may not accurately predict a responder, and that in certain circumstances the likelihood of success is so high that it is unnecessary. The author undertakes the trial procedure routinely, as this allows consideration of cases in whom clinical predictors of success are low.

In treating any form of chronic persistent pain it is important that a diagnosis is made. It is important that treatable conditions are not missed (e.g. unrecognized recurrent prolapse of disc following back surgery), and in addition one of the best predictive indicators for successful stimulation is the diagnostic category.

Some of these categories prove difficult to treat for technical reasons. For example it is difficult to achieve effective stimulation of midline areas such as the peri-anal area; however when stimulation is obtained pain relief can be excellent. Another problem in such cases is unwanted excessive stimulation in surrounding areas. Another area which is difficult to access is the head and neck, particularly the scalp.

Attention is also drawn to the failed back surgery syndrome. There continues to be enthusiasm for the treatment of the back pain elements of the condition by SCS although the success rate is poor; no trials exist to confirm efficacy. However SCS does prove effective for the leg pain elements of the condition.

Since it is a non-destructive technique it should be used in preference to destructive techniques (e.g. dorsal root entry zone lesions (DREZ)) even if the chance of success is less, since most destructive techniques have a high delayed relapse rate, and may cause neurological deficit. Consequently it is reasonable practice to perform a trial of SCS for brachial plexus avulsion pain (prior to DREZ). As a low-risk procedure, trial of SCS is worth considering as an alternative to destructive lesions for central post-stroke pain.

| Indication | Success rate |
| --- | --- |
| Angina<br>Ischaemic limb pain | Almost certain response |
| Causalgia, regional pain syndrome<br>Reflex sympathetic dystrophy<br>Peripheral nerve lesion*<br>Brachial plexus damage*<br>Cauda equina damage*<br>Nerve root avulsion*<br>Amputation stump pain | Success rate ≈ 70–80% |
| Painful diabetic peripheral neuropathy<br>Leg pain after Failed Back Surgery Syndrome<br>Back pain after Failed Back Surgery Syndrome<br>Arachnoiditis<br>Partial spinal cord lesion<br>Phantom limb pain<br>Post-herpetic neuralgia | Moderate success ≈ 40–50% |
| Nociceptive pain including cancer<br>Central post-stroke pain<br>Vaginal, penile and peri-anal pain<br>Intercostal neuralgia | Low chance of success |
| Facial anaesthesia dolorosa<br>Atypical facial pain<br>Complete cord lesion<br>Abdominal pain | Do not respond |

* If there is nerve injury with preserved, though disordered sensation (dysaesthesia) then success is likely; if there is established neurological deficit then response is unlikely.

## Case selection

It may be considered under three headings: diagnosis, influences on the pain and response to trial.

**1. *Diagnosis*** (as discussed above).

**2. *Influences on the pain.*** Most of these can be elucidated in the history in out-patients. If the pain is susceptible to external influence it is more likely to respond to spinal cord stimulation. Examples are the response of the pain to changes in temperature, to rubbing, to transcutaneous stimulation and to distraction. A reduction in pain indicates a high chance of stimulation being effective. Increase in pain due to allodynia can also predict a good response, though this is not as hopeful a predictor as when there is pain relief. Some practitioners use a test to provoke counter-irritation such as the injection of hypertonic saline into the interspinous ligament. This produces an intense local irritation; if this irritation substantially reduces or abolishes the pain then SCS is predicted to be effective. Using these clinical criteria, those with positive features produce an excellent outcome after permanent stimulation in approximately 60% of cases.

**3. *Response to trial.*** A positive response indicates a high likelihood of success, though not a certainty. In the audit referred to below a positive trial predicted a 90% chance of success (86% excellent outcomes); however it is not perfect and 10% of responders ultimately prove failures.

It can be seen that the percutaneous trial is particularly important in the groups where success is predicted to be 40–50% or less. SCS is one of a number of treatments that could be used for certain conditions, although it will be clear from the above that there are some conditions in which its use is indicated if less invasive treatments fail. Where the chance of success is small, there are as yet no clear criteria to direct the choice of therapy between say, SCS and other expensive and invasive procedures such as implantable intrathecal drug delivery systems. The author recommends extreme caution in assessing developments in this area.

## Outcome

In one series examining non-vascular indications for stimulation only 46% ultimately were implanted. 22% were rejected altogether (predicted to be poor responders), and 22% were treated in other ways (TNS, medical analgesics). 8% required a different surgical procedure (e.g. removal of recurrent disc) and 2% refused implantation. Out of the 88 cases implanted, 79 (90%) were adjudged successful (good or excellent pain relief) and 10% failures (poor relief or none) with a minimum follow-up of 1 year. Few studies exist showing long-term outcome. However, in series that do exist there is a reduction in success rate with time, although a reasonable expectation is that 75% of patients will experience more than a 50% reduction of their pain 5 years after implantation. There is often a difference of opinion between patient and doctor as to the efficacy of the treatment.

## Post-operative management and follow-up

Following successful implantation good results are obtained only when there is adequate follow-up. In the author's unit this is achieved by a specialist nurse and dedicated physiotherapist running 'neuromodulation clinics' with the implanting neurosurgeon. There should be support available from other pain specialists. Multi-disciplinary input is necessary for all but the most straightforward of cases. It may help to know that in many series the revision rate is quite high, anywhere between 25–50% of implants requiring surgical revision, and the use of battery-powered implantable devices means replacement will be required every 3–5 years. The fact that this is necessary is some demonstration of the long-term efficacy of the treatment.

## SCS for vascular disease: PVD, angina

SCS is extremely effective in treating these conditions. The action seems to be different from that of pure pain relief in that the mechanism appears to be an inhibition of the descending sympathetic pathway in the spinal cord. This is believed to prevent sympathetically mediated vasoconstriction. Supraspinal pathways are probably not involved and are certainly less important than in simple pain relief.

## Angina

SCS is effective in over 80% of cases. There is excellent pain relief, and the patient's usage of GTN declines. The inhibition of sympathetic vasoconstriction also appears to improve myocardial function, and it may be this that provides pain relief. At higher exercise levels the patients still experience angina, so this is not felt to be an unsafe treatment. In uncontrolled studies, survival seems to be improved compared with predictions from actuarial tables.

## PVD

SCS is highly effective in treating the pain of intermittent claudication due to peripheral vascular disease. It is more effective in the early stages of the disease. Increases in skin temperature, signals from laser-Doppler, and transcutaneous oxygen measurements occur with stimulation. This is a consequence of sympathetic system inhibition. There is, however, no evidence for an increase in muscle blood flow. Overall 80% of cases notice an improvement in pain control; 65% an improvement in walking distance and in 30% this improvement will be significant. These percentages improve if end-stage disease is excluded. Improvements in ulcer healing are also claimed and there may be a reduction in the amputation rate. Unlike the case of angina it appears that the effect on pain is separate from that on flow, as stimulating at higher levels in the spine (T8 vs T12) is still effective. SCS can help in vasospastic conditions such as Raynaud's disease. It is worth trying in diabetics although the response rate is not as good due to the multiplicity of problems, both vascular and neuropathic.

## Diabetic neuropathy

Painful diabetic neuropathy can be difficult to treat. However of ten patients assessed by trial stimulation eight responded at the trial stage and were implanted. Of these six obtained long-term relief ( >6 months); one did not and one died from an unrelated cause. There was relief of both the neuropathic pain and exercise tolerance.

## Multiple sclerosis

Approximately 25% of cases of multiple sclerosis experience some form of central pain syndrome. These syndromes may respond to SCS. An additional benefit is that improvements in bladder control may result in up to 70–80% of patients.

# Deep brain stimulation

### Indications

Severe chronic pain in face, arms or legs, often due to partial nerve injury such as may occur in amputation or stroke. It can be used in cases of central post-stroke pain. Many patients will be reluctant to undergo this form of surgery for a chronic pain condition; it is of course the case that any procedure invasive to the brain carries risk of stroke and to life, albeit very small. Invariably the patient will have found other methods – including trial of spinal cord stimulation to be ineffective.

## Methods

Under local anaesthetic a burr hole is made in the skull and an electrode passed stereotactically to the intended target, normally within the thalamus, though some have tried other sites such as peri-aqueductal grey matter. A trial of stimulation is then performed to make sure the electrode is in the desired physiological target, and then a trial of the therapeutic effect over a few days. After a few days, and provided the trial is successful, then a permanent device is implanted and connected to this electrode. The technique originally fell out of favour because of problems with electrode design but has been revisited recently with improvements in electrode design (mainly motivated by an increase in deep brain stimulation for movement disorders). A trial stage is required because a significant number of patients will turn out to be non-responders and a stimulator inappropriate.

## Outcomes

Perhaps only 50% of patients will respond and be implanted. The overall conclusion is that this technique is unproven.

# Motor cortex stimulation

## Indications

The main indication is for central post-stroke pain where the referred area in which the pain is felt comprises upper limb or face. The leg motor cortex is difficult to target being mainly in the interhemispheric fissure, as also is a large area; hence it cannot be considered when the syndrome covers half the sensorium.

## Methods

A craniotomy is performed and electrodes placed over the motor cortex. Intra-operative neurophysiology and/or sophisticated image guidance techniques may be necessary to locate the part of the brain which is the motor cortex. In the author's unit the practice now is to obtain a functional MRI scan in which the motor cortex has been localized; to employ intraoperative frameless stereotactic neuronavigation techniques to facilitate placement of an electrode. The final placement is confirmed by neurophysiological methods – direct motor cortex stimulation and recording of the somatosensory evoked response. A trial is performed before a permanent device is used, as the percentage of patients who turn out to be responsive to this form of therapy is small. If the cortex is stimulated too vigorously there is a risk of seizures. Unlike stimulation of the sensory pathways there are no paraesthesiae to indicate function of the stimulator, so over-stimulation is a real risk. Since it is an intracranial procedure there must also be risk of stroke (and therefore to life) from haemorrhage or infection and a risk of epilepsy, however low these risks must be.

## Outcomes

These have not been uniformly encouraging so currently the method should be regarded as unproven. However using the technology mentioned above it has been possible to more accurately and reliably target the motor cortex, which has led in turn to more optimistic reports in the literature. It has been realized with the advent of functional MRI that there is sufficient plasticity of the nervous system that the position of the motor cortex may not be as predicted anatomically following stroke. However, there is impetus behind development of such techniques as they represent an option of medical management for a minority of patients who have failed all other treatments. Such 'heroic' techniques must however be considered in the light of all the other factors contributing to the experience of pain in this vulnerable group of patients.

## Further reading

Jacobs MJ, Jorning PJ, Beckers RC, Ubbink DT, van Kleef M, Slaaf DW, Reneman RS. Foot salvage and improvement of microvascular blood flow as a result of epidural spinal cord electrical stimulation. *Journal of Vascular Surgery*, 1990; **12**: 354–60.

North RB, Roark GL. Spinal cord stimulation for chronic pain. *Neurosurgery Clinics of North America*, 1995; **6**: 145–55.

North RB, Kidd DH, Zahurak M, James CS, Long DM. Spinal cord stimulation for chronic, intractable pain: experience over two decades. *Neurosurgery*, 1993; **32**(3): 384–95.

Rees G. Mechanism of action of spinal cord stimulation. *Pain Reviews*, 1994; **1**: 184–98.

Simpson BA. Spinal cord stimulation. *Pain Reviews*, 1994; **1**: 199–230.

## Related topics of interest

# THERAPY – TENS, ACUPUNCTURE AND LASER STIMULATION

*Kate Grady*

## Transcutaneous electrical nerve stimulation (TENS)

The transcutaneous electrical stimulation of peripheral nerves through intact skin is effective in controlling some pains. This is achieved by the placement of two electrodes over the painful area and the passage of a small current through the electrodes. The current is generated from a portable battery-operated device. Stimulation of low-threshold afferents (Aβ mechano-ceptors) causes inhibition of the passage of high-threshold pain fibre impulses (Aδ and C fibres) at spinal cord level. High-frequency current selectively stimulates larger afferent fibres. It may also increase the refractory period and reduce firing rate in smaller afferent pain fibres. Low-frequency stimulation (Aδ mechanism) can produce analgesia in patients who have failed to respond to the more conventional high-frequency stimulation. This is thought to work by activating inhibitory descending neuronal influence in the dorsal horn of the spinal cord.

### Uses

A systematic review has shown TENS to reduce pain and improve the range of movement in chronic low-back pain patients. In osteoarthritis of knee, TENS and acupuncture like TENS were significantly better than placebo in reducing pain and knee stiffness. A trial of TENS is appropriate for most pains which have some noci-ceptive. Its success in the treatment of central pain depends on whether dorsal columns and medial lemniscal pathways are intact. TENS can treat the pain of mild post-herpetic neuralgia. Where afferent fibre destruction is extensive it may aggra-vate the pain. TENS has been effective in facial pain, myofascial pain, mechanical back pain, post-amputation pain, refractory angina and peripheral nerve injury, particularly when there is paraesthesia. TENS can be effective in visceral, neuro-pathic or metastatic pain of cancer. Twenty-five per cent of radicular pain responds to TENS.

### Practicalities

Electrode pads are made of a size which minimizes current density. Good contact with skin is necessary and is achieved by adhesiveness of the pads or the application of conducting gel underneath the pads. TENS should be used for at least 30 minutes at a time. It can be used for longer periods. Some patients gain relief only for the period that the machine is in use. Others feel relief beyond the period of use. Sites of application should be rotated to avoid skin irritation. TENS should not be used whilst asleep or whilst driving. Electrode pads are applied to the painful area. They should not be applied to an insensate area. For the treatment of radicular pain elec-trode pads are placed over the dermatomal distribution of the affected root. Elec-trodes should not be placed on the anterior surface of the neck, lest they affect the carotid sinus. Constant high-frequency stimulation is the normal mode of use, most patients preferring a rate of 40–70 Hz. Those who fail to get relief from this mode may respond to stimulation at a frequency of 2–4 Hz. This requires a higher intensity and may cause uncomfortable muscle contractions. Some machines therefore have a modulation facility which allows switching of current and frequency at short intervals.

## Limitations

TENS is relatively safe with few side-effects. It should not be used in pregnancy until the onset of labour. It should not be used in the patient with a cardiac pacemaker. Side-effects are limited to skin irritation and scorching under the pads. This may be severe if electrode pads have wrongly been applied to an insensate area. Patients may encounter difficulty in placing electrodes at awkward sites.

# Acupuncture

Acupuncture is an ancient Chinese medical art which has gained momentum in the West over the past 25 years. Traditionally the understanding of mechanism was based on the concept that the body requires a balance of energy factors to be in good health. The balance of the energy factors, Yin and Yang was thought to be restored by acupuncture. Energy flowing along intangible meridians to and from vital organs was believed to be effected by sharp objects applied at certain points along the meridians. The rationale of acupuncture in Western medical practice is that high-threshold mechanoceptors are activated by low-frequency high-intensity stimulation. They in turn affect descending inhibition in the spinal cord.

Electroacupuncture is the augmentation of the mechanical needle stimulus by using electricity.

## Uses

The use of acupuncture has many enthusiasts, in conventional medical practice, other disciplines such as physiotherapy and in the hands of complementary acupuncture therapists, and is a widely used modality for the treatment of many pains. However, the evidence for its effectiveness, as assessed by randomized controlled trials has not been shown. Recent proposals to have the technique widely available have been based predominantly on the results of observational studies, rather than these trials. Controlled studies involve techniques such as 'sham' acupuncture, where needles are placed without reference to specific acupuncture points, and ideally should be independently evaluated. This is not to say that acupuncture 'does not work', rather that the evidence is unavailable at the present time. The difficulty of assessing the response and integrating the practice of acupuncture into current practice is establishing the length of time that symptom relief may be obtained and the extent to which other treatments undertaken simultaneously may be contributing to the overall effect.

## Practicalities

Asepsis is important and needles should not be positioned in infected-looking areas. Needles should be carefully placed to avoid the complications of pneumothorax, cardiac tamponade, damage to nervous tissue or the piercing of blood vessels.

## Limitations

Improvement is short-term and repeated treatments are necessary to sustain pain relief. However, as with other passive short-term treatments, the attendant risks are patient request for treatment which outstrips resources and no improvement of function. Acupuncture has to be incorporated into an overall strategy of pain management.

## Laser

High-powered lasers are used in surgery and exert their effect by generating heat in body tissues. The non-thermal application of laser energy has a tissue effect which is important and its first potential beneficial effect was described in wound healing. Low-level laser therapy (LLLT) has been suggested to be useful in a wide variety of painful musculoskeletal pain conditions and in post-herpetic neuralgia. The precise mechanism is unknown but it is suggested that the primary response takes place at cellular level and consists of increased microvasculature flow, improved lymphatic drainage, with increased macrophage and fibroblast activity and collagen synthesis to improve healing. The secondary phase comprises the release of endorphins, enkephalins and prostaglandins which have antinociceptive effect.

## Uses

LLLT has been used in the treatment of many painful conditions such as post-traumatic pain of the vertebral column and limbs, chronic post-surgical pains, failed back surgery syndrome, and musculoskeletal pains without radiological evidence of gross skeletal deformity or damage. Systematic review of its use in osteoarthritis suggested more consistent methodology of application is needed to assess effect. In rheumatoid arthritis, a systematic review suggests it should be considered for short-term relief of pain and morning stiffness. It has been shown to reduce both intensity and distribution of pain in post-herpetic neuralgia of at least six months duration and unresponsive to other methods of treatment.

## Limitations

LLLT is not associated with any adverse reactions or troublesome side-effects.

## Further reading

Alexander JR, Macdonald T, Coates W. The discovery of transcutaneous spinal electroanalgesia and its relief of chronic pain. *Physiotherapy*, 1995; **81**(11): 653–61.
Ernst E, White A. Acupuncture: safety first. *British Medical Journal*, 1997; **314:** 1362.

## Systematic reviews

Brosseau L, Welch V, Wells G. *Low level laser therapy for treating osteoarthritis (Cochrane review)*. In: The Cochrane Library, Issue 4, 2000. Oxford: Update software.
Brosseau L, Welch V, Wells G. *Low level laser therapy for treating rheumatoid arthritis (Cochrane review)*. In: The Cochrane Library, Issue 4, 2000. Oxford: Update software.

Ernst E, White AR. Acupuncture for back pain: a metaanalysis of randomized controlled trials. *Archives of Internal Medicine*, 1998; **158:** 2235–41.

Ezzo J *et al.* Is acupuncture effective for the treatment of chronic pain? A systematic review. *Pain*, 2000; **86:** 217–225.

Gadsby JG, Flowerdew MW. The effectiveness of transcutaneous electrical nerve stimulation (TENS) and acupuncture-like transcutaneous electrical nerve stimulation (ALTENS) in the treatment of patients with chronic low back pain. In: Bombardier C, Natchemson A, Deyo R, de Bie R, Bouter L, Shekelle P, Waddell G, Roland M (eds). *The Cochrane Collaboration Issue 1.* Oxford: The Cochrane Library, 1997.

## Related topic of interest

Nociceptive pain – an overview (p. 117).

# INDEX

Phantom pain, 115, 125, 130–132, 145, 154, 174, 201

Physiotherapy, 33, 65, 71, 93, 98, 100, 105, 124, 136, 139, 193–194, 196, 207

Psychological factors, 18, 25, 26, 35, 43, 47, 65, 69, 73, 74, 75, 77, 78, 89, 92, 99, 102, 115, **125–127,** 129, 130, 136, 149, 151, 180, 188–189, 192, **195–196**

Psychosocial assessment, 17, 18, 25–28, 31, 63, 75, 97, 99, 129–130

Radiofrequency, 5, 36, 37, 38, 54, 69, 85, 93, 100, 101, 109, 110, 111, 112, 120, 142, 179, **181,** 184, 186

Reflex sympathetic dystrophy, *see* complex regional pain syndrome

Sciatic stretch test, 21, 30

Sciatica, 40, 41, 42, 139, 183

Self-help groups, 3

Self-rating questionnaires, 17, 26, 73, 195

Sensitization, 47–48, 80, 104, 106, **114–115,** 118, 119, 126, 131, 134, 143, 147, 162, 176, 181, 189

Shoulder pain, 95, 97, 99, 130, 145, 151, 167, 180

Somatization disorder, 75

Spinal cord
    injury, 54, 69, 91, **147–149,** 169, 177, 184–185, 187, 201
    stimulation, 43–44, 64, 93, 183, 185, **198–204**

Spinal stenosis, 30, 41, **42**

Stereotactic surgery, 111, 183, 204

Stroke, 45, 69, 77, 95, 110, 113, **150–152,** 167, 200–205

Sudeck's atrophy, *see* complex regional pain

syndrome

Suicide, 26, 73, 134

Sympathectomy, intravenous guanethidine, *see* drugs, guanethidine

Symptoms
    fever, 29
    morning stiffness, 29
    night-time pain, 29
    sphincter disturbance, 29–30, 53, 96, 208

Syndrome
    Brown Sequard, 147
    burning mouth, 80–81
    carpal tunnel, 105, 140, 145
    chronic fatigue, 197
    complex regional pain, **67–72,** 96, 105, 113, 148, 154, 158, 167, 174, 176
    CPPWOP, **125**
    irritable bowel, 80–81, 127, 197
    loin pain/haematuria, 127
    Pancoast, 185

Syringomyelia, 44, 45, 147, 148

Thalamic pain, *see* central post-stroke pain

Thoracotomy, 144, **145,** 159

Tolerance, 59, 137, 169, 189, **190**

Transcutaneous electrical nerve stimulation, 18, 64, 78, 87, 121, 132, 148, **206–207**

Transdermal delivery of drugs, *see* fentanyl

Vitamins, 81, 105

Vulvodynia, **128–129**

Whiplash, **99–100**

Windup, 47, **114,** 119, 173